Checkpoint Controls and Cancer

METHODS IN MOLECULAR BIOLOGY™

John M. Walker, SERIES EDITOR

METHODS IN MOLECULAR BIOLOGY™

Checkpoint Controls and Cancer

Volume 1
Reviews and Model Systems

Edited by

Axel H. Schönthal, PhD

*Department of Molecular Microbiology and Immunology
and K. Norris Jr. Comprehensive Cancer Center,
University of Southern California Keck School of Medicine,
Los Angeles, CA*

HUMANA PRESS ✳ TOTOWA, NEW JERSEY

© 2004 Humana Press Inc.
999 Riverview Drive, Suite 208
Totowa, New Jersey 07512

www.humanapress.com

This publication is printed on acid-free paper. ∞
ANSI Z39.48-1984 (American Standards Institute)
Permanence of Paper for Printed Library Materials.

Production Editor: Tracy Catanese

Cover illustration: Figure 3 from Volume 1, Chapter 12, "Methods for Analyzing Checkpoint Responses in *Caenorhabditis elegans*," by Anton Gartner, Amy J. MacQueen, and Anne M. Villeneuve.

Cover design by Patricia F. Cleary.

For additional copies, pricing for bulk purchases, and/or information about other Humana titles, contact Humana at the above address or at any of the following numbers: Tel.: 973-256-1699; Fax: 973-256-8341; E-mail: humana@humanapr.com; or visit our website: www.humanapress.com

Printed in the United States of America. 10 9 8 7 6 5 4 3 2 1

1-59259-788-2 (e-book)
ISSN 1064-3745

Library of Congress Cataloging in Publication Data

Checkpoint controls and cancer / edited by Axel H. Schönthal.
    p. cm. -- (Methods in molecular biology ; 280-281)
  Includes bibliographical references and index.
  Contents: V. 1. Reviews and model systems -- v. 2. Activation and regulation protocols.
  ISBN 1-58829-214-2 (v. 1 : alk. paper) -- ISBN 1-58829-500-1 (v. 2 : alk. paper)
    1. Carcinogenesis--Laboratory manuals. 2. Cellular signal transduction--Laboratory manuals. 3. Cellular control mechanisms--Laboratory manuals. I. Schönthal, Axel H. II. Series.

RC268.5.C48 2004
616.99'4071--dc22

                                                                    2004040578

Preface

Intracellular checkpoint controls constitute a network of signal transduction pathways that protect cells from external stresses and internal errors. External stresses can be generated by the continuous assault of DNA-damaging agents, such as environmental mutagens, ultraviolet (UV) light, ionizing radiation, or the reactive oxygen species that can arise during normal cellular metabolism. In response to any of these assaults on the integrity of the genome, the activation of the network of checkpoint control pathways can lead to diverse cellular responses, such as cell cycle arrest, DNA repair, or elimination of the cell by cell death (apoptosis) if the damage cannot be repaired. Moreover, internal errors can occur during the highly orchestrated replication of the cellular genome and its distribution into daughter cells. Here, the temporal order of these cell cycle events must be strictly enforced—for example, to ensure that DNA replication is complete and occurs only once before cell division, or to monitor mitotic spindle assembly, and to prevent exit from mitosis until chromosome segregation has been completed. Thus, well functioning checkpoint mechanisms are central to the maintenance of genomic integrity and the basic viability of cells and, therefore, are essential for proper development and survival.

The importance of proper functioning of checkpoints becomes plainly obvious under conditions in which this control network malfunctions and fails. Depending on the severity and timing, failure of this machinery can lead to embryonic lethality, genetic diseases, and cancer. Cancer in particular has been recognized as a disease in which acquired mutations and loss of genomic integrity decidedly contribute to its origination and progression. Most, if not all, cancer cells exhibit incomplete or malfunctioning checkpoint control pathways, which constitutes a situation that is further aggravated because this absence of efficient controls allows for even more deleterious mutations to accumulate. The enhanced potential of cancer cells to survive under suboptimal conditions and their increasing ability to withstand chemotherapeutic intervention are but two of the consequences. Thus, identifying the molecular components of checkpoint controls and understanding the complexity of their spaciotemporal interactions is a major goal of current cancer research. Besides satisfying our academic curiosity, novel insights and advances in this complex area are essential for the development of new and more effective therapies.

Experts from 10 different countries have contributed their detailed knowledge to the present two-volume work, *Checkpoint Controls and Cancer*, which presents a collection of indispensable tools and their applications that will further advance our understanding of the intricacies of checkpoint controls. Each volume is divided into two parts. Part I of *Volume 1: Reviews and Model Systems* contains comprehensive review articles that introduce all of the important components of checkpoint controls, describe their intricate interactions, and highlight the relevance of these processes to the cancer problem. Here, the amazing complexities of checkpoint controls—and the gaps that exist in our knowledge thereof—become distinctly apparent. Part II illustrates the advantages of utilizing diverse model systems, such as intact human skin or knockout mice, as well as other most useful organisms, such as *Xenopus, Drosophila, Caenorhabditis*, and yeast. As has been shown time and again, the convergence of information from various model systems is able to crossfertilize and accelerate research both across disciplines and beyond the boundaries of a particular species. This is especially true for the study of yeast, which has already provided major insights into the function of cell cycle and checkpoint controls. *Volume 2: Activation and Regulation Protocols* is a collection of "how-to" chapters with stepwise instructions that focuses on the individual components of checkpoint controls and describes the detailed analysis of their activity. Part II completes this collection by providing various experimental approaches for the manipulation of checkpoint pathways and the analysis of the resulting consequences for the cellular phenotype. Altogether, this collection of protocols and proven techniques will be useful for all researchers, whether they be novices who need step-by-step instructions, or experienced scientists who want to explore new approaches or model systems for the study of checkpoint controls and cancer.

I would like to thank the authors for the clear and detailed descriptions of the procedures they provided, and for the many useful hints they included in the notes section to each chapter. Those authors who provided general review chapters are thanked for their thoughtful and nicely structured presentation of their topics and some marvelous illustrations. I wish to acknowledge John Walker, the series editor, for his support, and the staff at Humana Press who helped produce this volume.

Axel H. Schönthal

Contents of Volume 1

vii

CONTENTS OF THE COMPANION VOLUME

Volume 2: Activation and Regulation Protocols

Contributors

ROBERT T. ABRAHAM • Program in Signal Transduction Research, The Burnham Institute, La Jolla, CA

PETER D. ADAMS • Department of Basic Science, Fox Chase Cancer Center, Philadelphia, PA

GENEVIÈVE ALMOUZNI • Research Section, Institut Curie, Paris, France

PAUL R. ANDREASSEN • Institut de Biologie Structurale J.-P. Ebel (CEA-CNRS-UJF), Grenoble, France

STEVEN P. ANGUS • Department of Molecular Genetics and Microbiology, Duke University Medical Center, Durham, NC

HEATHER BEAMISH • Centre for Immunology and Cancer Research, University of Queensland, Princess Alexandra Hospital, Brisbane, Queensland, Australia

MOURAD BENDJENNAT • Institut de Biologie Structurale J.-P. Ebel (CEA-CNRS-UJF), Grenoble, France

NORBERT BERNDT • Division of Hematology/Oncology, Children's Hospital Los Angeles, Los Angeles, CA

EMILY E. BOSCO • Department of Cell Biology, Vontz Center for Molecular Studies, University of Cincinnati College of Medicine, Cincinnati, OH

ERIC J. BROWN • Department of Cancer Biology, Abramson Family Cancer Research Institute, University of Pennsylvania School of Medicine, Philadelphia, PA

DANIEL J. BURKE • Department of Biochemistry and Molecular Genetics, University of Virginia Medical Center, Charlottesville, VA

NELLY BURON • INSERM U517, IFR100, Faculty of Medicine, Dijon, France

SÉVERINE CATHELIN • INSERM U517, IFR100, Faculty of Medicine, Dijon, France

JUNJIE CHEN • Department of Oncology, Mayo Clinic, Rochester, MN

GARY G. CHIANG • Program in Signal Transduction Research, The Burnham Institute, La Jolla, CA

VINCENZO COSTANZO • Department of Genetics and Development, Columbia University, New York, NY

KATHLEEN D. DANENBERG • Response Genetics Inc., Los Angeles, CA

PETER V. DANENBERG • Department of Molecular Biology and Biochemistry and K. Norris Jr. Comprehensive Cancer Center, University of Southern California, Keck School of Medicine, Los Angeles, CA

ZBIGNIEW DARZYNKIEWICZ • *Brander Cancer Research Institute at New York Medical Center, Hawthorne, NY*

BIPIN C. DASH • *Laboratory of Molecular Oncology and Cell Cycle Regulation, Howard Hughes Medical Institute, and Departments of Medicine, Genetics, and Pharmacology and Abramson Cancer Center, University of Pennsylvania School of Medicine, Philadelphia, PA*

CHU-XIA DENG • *Genetics of Development and Disease Branch, Digestive and Kidney Diseases, National Cancer Institute, National Institutes of Health, Bethesda, MD*

WAFIK EL-DEIRY • *Laboratory of Molecular Oncology and Cell Cycle Regulation, Howard Hughes Medical Institute, and Departments of Medicine, Genetics, and Pharmacology and Abramson Cancer Center, University of Pennsylvania School of Medicine, Philadelphia, PA*

GUOWEI FANG • *Department of Biological Sciences, Stanford University, Stanford, CA*

RODOLPHE FILOMENKO • *INSERM U517, IFR100, Faculty of Medicine, Dijon, France*

ARUN FOTEDAR • *Sidney Kimmel Cancer Center, San Diego, CA*

RATI FOTEDAR • *Institut de Biologie Structurale J.-P. Ebel (CEA-CNRS-UJF), Grenoble, France*

BRIAN G. GABRIELLI • *Centre for Immunology and Cancer Research, University of Queensland, Princess Alexandra Hospital, Brisbane, Queensland, Australia*

ANTON GARTNER • *Department of Cell Biology, Max Planck Institute for Biochemistry, Martinsried, Germany*

JEAN GAUTIER • *Department of Genetics and Development, Columbia University, New York, NY*

KATRINA E. GORDON • *Beatson Institute for Cancer Research, Glasgow, Scotland*

CATHERINE M. GREEN • *Genome Damage and Stability Centre, University of Sussex, Brighton, UK*

NURI GUEVEN • *The Queensland Institute of Medical Research, PO Royal Brisbane Hospital, Herston, Queensland, Australia*

INGO HASSEPASS • *Cell Cycle Control and Carcinogenesis, German Cancer Research Center (DKFZ), Heidelberg, Germany*

INGRID HOFFMAN • *Department of Applied Tumorvirology, Cell Cycle Control and Carcinogenesis (F045), German Cancer Research Center (DKFZ), Heidelberg, Germany*

BURNLEY JAKLEVIC • *Molecular, Cellular, and Developmental Biology, University of Colorado, Boulder, CO*

DONGMIN KANG • *Department of Biological Sciences, Stanford University, Stanford, CA*

MICHAEL B. KASTAN • *Department of Hematology-Oncology, St. Jude Children's Research Hospital, Memphis, TN*

ERIK S. KNUDSEN • *Department of Cell Biology, Vontz Center for Molecular Studies, University of Cincinnati College of Medicine, Cincinnati, OH*

SERGEI KOZLOV • *The Queensland Institute of Medical Research, Royal Brisbane Hospital, Herston, Queensland, Australia*

MARTIN F. LAVIN • *The Queensland Cancer Fund Research Unit, The Queensland Institute of Medical Research, Royal Brisbane Hospital, Herston, Queensland, Australia*

SUXING LIU • *Tumor Biology Department, Schering-Plough Research Institute, Kenilworth, NJ*

EMMANUELLE LOGETTE • *INSERM U517, IFR100, Faculty of Medicine, Dijon, France*

ZHENKUN LOU • *Department of Oncology, Mayo Clinic, Rochester, MN*

NOEL F. LOWNDES • *Department of Biochemistry and National Centre for Biomedical Engineering Science, National University of Ireland Galway, Galway, Ireland*

JOHN W. LUDLOW • *Vesta Therapeutics, Research Triangle Park, NC*

AMY J. MACQUEEN • *Department of Molecular Biology, UT Southwestern Medical Center, Dallas, TX*

ROBERT L. MARGOLIS • *Institut de Biologie Structurale J.-P. Ebel (CEA-CNRS-UJF), Grenoble, France*

CHRISTOPHER N. MAYHEW • *Department of Cell Biology, Vontz Center for Molecular Studies, University of Cincinnati College of Medicine, Cincinnati, OH*

JILL A. MELLO • *Research Section, Institut Curie, UMR218 du Centre National de la Recherche Scientifique (CNRS), Paris, France*

ASRA MIRZA • *Tumor Biology Department, Schering-Plough Research Institute, Kenilworth, NJ*

JONATHAN G. MOGGS • *Research Section, Institut Curie, UMR218 du Centre National de la Recherche Scientifique (CNRS), Paris, France*

DAVID M. NELSON • *Department of Basic Science, Fox Chase Cancer Center, Philadelphia, PA*

HIROSHI NOJIMA • *Department of Molecular Genetics, Research Institute for Microbial Diseases, Osaka University, Suita, Osaka, Japan*

E. KENNETH PARKINSON • *Beatson Institute for Cancer Research, Garscube Estate, Bearsden, Glasgow, Scotland*

SANDRA PAVEY • *Queensland Institute of Medical Research, PO Royal Brisbane Hospital, Brisbane, Queensland, Australia*

STÉPHANIE PLENCHETTE • *INSERM U517, IFR100, Faculty of Medicine, Dijon, France*

MAXIM POUSTOVOITOV • *Department of Basic Science, Fox Chase Cancer Center, Philadelphia, PA*

PIOTR POZAROWSKI • *Department of Clinical Immunology, School of Medicine, Lublin, Poland*

ENNIO PROSPERI • *Istituto di Genetica Molecolare del CNR, sez. Istochimica e Citometria, Pavia, Italy*

AMANDA PURDY • *Molecular, Cellular, and Developmental Biology, University of Colorado, Boulder, CO*

KIRSTEN ROBERTSON • *Department of Genetics and Development, Columbia University, New York, NY*

DENNIS SALONGA • *Response Genetics Inc., Los Angeles, CA*

HIDELITA SANTOS • *Department of Basic Science, Fox Chase Cancer Center, Philadelphia, PA*

HIDEYUKI SAYA • *Department of Tumor Genetics and Biology, Graduate School of Medical Sciences, Kumamoto University, Honjo, Kumamoto, Japan*

SYLKE SCHNEIDER • *Department of Molecular Biology and Biochemistry and K. Norris Jr. Comprehensive Cancer Center, University of Southern California Keck School of Medicine, Los Angeles, CA*

AXEL H. SCHÖNTHAL • *Department of Molecular Microbiology and Immunology and K. Norris Jr. Comprehensive Cancer Center, University of Southern California Keck School of Medicine, Los Angeles, CA*

SHAUN P. SCOTT • *The Queensland Institute of Medical Research, Royal Brisbane Hospital, Herston, Queensland, Australia*

DIMITRIOS A. SKOUFIAS • *Institut de Biologie Structurale J.-P. Ebel (CEA-CNRS-UJF), Grenoble, France*

ERIC SOLARY • *INSERM U517, IFR100, Faculty of Medicine, Dijon, France*

STÉPHANIE SOLIER • *INSERM U517, IFR100, Faculty of Medicine, Dijon, France*

DAVID A. SOLOMON • *Department of Cell Biology, Vontz Center for Molecular Studies, University of Cincinnati College of Medicine, Cincinnati, OH*

GEORGE R. STARK • *Department of Molecular Biology, Lerner Research Institute, The Cleveland Clinic Foundation, Cleveland, OH*

DAVID F. STERN • Department of Pathology, School of Medicine, Yale University, New Haven, CT

LUCIA A. STIVALA • Dipartimento di Medicina Sperimentale, sez. Patologia Generale "C. Golgi," Università di Pavia, Pavia, Italy

P. TODD STUKENBERG • Department of Biochemistry and Molecular Genetics, University of Virginia Medical Center, Charlottesville, VA

TIN TIN SU • Molecular, Cellular, and Developmental Biology, University of Colorado, Boulder, CO

VALERY SUDAKIN • Institute for Cancer Research, The Fox Chase Cancer Center, Philadelphia, PA

TAMOTSU SUDO • Department of Tumor Genetics and Biology, Graduate School of Medical Sciences, Kumamoto University, Honjo, Kumamoto, Japan

ZHANYUN TANG • Department of Pharmacology, UT Southwestern Medical Center, Dallas, TX

WILLIAM R. TAYLOR • Department of Biological Sciences, University of Toledo, Toledo, OH

KAZUMI UCHIDA • Department of Molecular Biology and Biochemistry and K. Norris Jr. Comprehensive Cancer Center, University of Southern California Keck School of Medicine, Los Angeles, CA

NAOTO T. UENO • Department of Blood and Marrow Transplantation, The University of Texas M. D. Anderson Cancer Center, Houston, TX

ANNE M. VILLENEUVE • Departments of Developmental Biology and Genetics, Stanford University School of Medicine, Stanford, CA

HONGYAN WANG • Department of Radiation Oncology, Kimmel Cancer Center of Jefferson Medical College, Thomas Jefferson University, Philadelphia, PA

LUQUAN WANG • Discovery Technology Department, Schering-Plough Research Institute, Kenilworth, NJ

YA WANG • Department of Radiation Oncology, Kimmel Cancer Center of Jefferson Medical College, Thomas Jefferson University, Philadelphia, PA

ROBYN WARRENER • Centre for Immunology and Cancer Research, University of Queensland, Princess Alexandra Hospital, Brisbane, Queensland, Australia

JIM WONG • Department of Biological Sciences, Stanford University, Stanford, CA

BO XU • Department of Genetics and Stanley S. Scott Cancer Center, Louisiana State University Health Sciences Center, New Orleans, LA

XIAOLING XU • Genetics of Development and Disease Branch, National Institute of Diabetes, Digestive and Kidney Diseases, National Cancer Institute, National Institutes of Health, Bethesda, MD

Xingzhi Xu • *Department of Pathology, Yale University School of Medicine, New Haven, CT*

Xiafen Ye • *Department of Basic Science, Fox Chase Cancer Center, Philadelphia, PA*

Christopher M. Yellman • *Department of Biochemistry and Molecular Genetics, University of Virginia Medical Center, Charlottesville, VA*

Tim J. Yen • *Institute for Cancer Research, The Fox Chase Cancer Center, Philadelphia, PA*

Ji Min Yochim • *Department of Molecular Biology and Biochemistry and K. Norris Jr. Comprehensive Cancer Center, University of Southern California, Keck School of Medicine, Los Angeles, CA*

Hongtao Yu • *Department of Pharmacology, UT Southwestern Medical Center, Dallas, TX*

I

Reviews of Checkpoint Controls, Their Involvement in the Development of Cancer, and Approaches to Their Investigation

1

G1 and S-Phase Checkpoints, Chromosome Instability, and Cancer

Hiroshi Nojima

Summary

Mitogen-dependent progression through the first gap phase (G1) of the mammalian cell-division cycle is precisely regulated so that normal cell division is coordinated with cell growth, while the initiation of DNA synthesis (S phase) is precisely ordered to prevent inappropriate amplification of the DNA that may cause genome instability. To ensure that these fundamental requirements of cell division are met, cells have developed a surveillance mechanism based on an intricate network of protein kinase signaling pathways that lead to several different types of checkpoints. Since these checkpoints are central to the maintenance of the genomic integrity and basic viability of the cells, defects in these pathways may result in either tumorigenesis or apoptosis, depending on the severity and nature of the defects. This review summarizes the genetic and molecular mechanisms of checkpoint activation in the G1/S and S phases of the mammalian cell cycle that monitor DNA damage and replication. The relevance of these mechanisms to the origin of cancer is also discussed.

Key Words: Cell cycle; checkpoints; G1/S; DNA damage; chromosome; p53; MYC; CHK1; CHK2; ATM; ATR; pRB; E2F; p21; INK4a; CDK2; Cyclin E; Cyclin G; NBS1; MRE11; BRCA1; MDM2; ARF; Cdc25A.

1. Introduction

Eukaryotic cells have developed a complex network of cell cycle checkpoint pathways. These act as surveillance mechanisms that ensure the proper progression of the cell cycle after exposure to various environmental stresses or after the occurrence of spontaneous perturbations such as DNA damage and improper progression of DNA replication *(1–4)*. These evolutionarily conserved surveillance mechanisms ensure that DNA replication remains faithful, thus guaranteeing the transmission of an unaltered genome and promoting the survival of the cells. The checkpoint regulatory machineries that serve as the guardians of proper cell cycle progression fulfill four fundamental consecutive

From: *Methods in Molecular Biology, vol. 280: Checkpoint Controls and Cancer, Volume 1: Reviews and Model Systems*
Edited by: Axel H. Schönthal © Humana Press Inc., Totowa, NJ

tasks. First, upon stress, they rapidly induce cell cycle arrest or delay. They then help activate the mechanisms that repair damaged DNA or stalled replication. They also maintain the cell cycle arrest until repair is complete. At this point, they then actively re-initiate cell cycle progression. The cell cycle arrest that is induced and maintained by these checkpoints gives the cell time not only to repair the cellular damage but also to wait for the dissipation of an exogenous cellular stress signal or to probe the availability of essential growth factors, hormones, or nutrients.

The cell cycle checkpoints were initially defined as constituting a regulatory mechanism that acts to arrest the cell cycle in response to DNA damage, so that cell cycle progression and repair could be temporally coordinated *(5,6)*. However, more recent work suggests that the checkpoints may play many more regulatory roles in various cellular events *(6)*. Indeed, they are now believed to regulate the transcription of DNA damage response genes *(7)*, the telomere length and chromatin structure *(8)*, the recruitment of proteins to damage sites *(2,3)*, the kinetochore attachment to spindle microtubules *(9)*, the arrangement of the cytoskeleton *(10,11)*, meiotic recombination *(12,13)*, meiotic chromosome pairing and segregation *(14)*, and the cell cycle timing in the first cell divisions of the embryo *(15)*. Notably, the checkpoint signaling pathways can also result in the activation of programmed cell death if cellular damage cannot be properly repaired *(16–19)*.

The stability of the genome is under constant threat from chemicals, radiation, and normal DNA metabolism. Therefore, if the checkpoints are not properly controlled, the cells may suffer potentially catastrophic DNA damage that can lead to elevated mutation rates, chromosome instability, and aneuploidy, all of which can contribute to tumorigenesis *(20)*. Failure of the G1/S phase and S-phase checkpoints to act properly is particularly deleterious because it may directly elicit chromosomal aberrations and the accumulation of deleterious mutations, which increase the likelihood of the occurrence of genetic syndromes and diseases such as cancer *(21,4)*. In this review, I will discuss the recent progress in the study of the mammalian checkpoints at the G1 and S phases that guard the entry into and the progression through the S phase and thereby ensure proper DNA replication. Occasionally studies on budding yeast, fission yeast, and other eukaryotes will be mentioned if their observations aid our understanding of mammalian checkpoint mechanisms. I will also focus on the evidence that supports the notion that aberrant checkpoint regulatory mechanisms may promote the incidence of DNA alterations that may lead to cancer.

2. Molecular Mechanism Controlling the G1/S Transition of Mammalian Cells

2.1. Factors Regulating G1 Phase of the Cell Cycle

2.1.1. G1 Phase CDK/Cyclin Complexes

The progression through the cell cycle is governed by the periodic activation and inactivation of cyclin-dependent kinase (CDK) complexes. The CDK proteins are Ser/Thr protein kinases, and their kinase activities are controlled by their association partners, which are called cyclins *(22)*. The protein levels of the CDKs remain constant through the cell cycle, whereas the levels of the cyclins vary during the cell cycle, owing to periodic expression and degradation. The timely regulation of different CDK/cyclin complexes is responsible for well-organized cell cycle progression, as these complexes act in G1 to initiate S phase and in G2 to initiate mitosis. These mechanisms are conserved from yeast to mammals *(23)*. The kinase activity of the CDKs is also tightly controlled by the binding of inhibitors and phosphorylation events.

In the middle of the cyclin proteins is a domain of well-conserved amino acid sequences called the *cyclin box*. While cyclins were originally characterized as being the regulatory subunit of CDK that is periodically expressed and degraded during the cell cycle *(24)*, it was later found that many cyclins do not cycle and that they can regulate cellular functions other than the cell cycle *(25)*. These include: cyclin G *(26)*, which is a regulatory subunit of protein phosphatase 1A *(27)*; cyclin H, which forms a complex with CDK7 that regulates not only other CDKs as a CDK-activating kinase (CAK) *(28)* but also transcription and DNA repair *(29)*; cyclin L, which is a regulatory subunit of CDK11 and promotes pre-mRNA splicing *(30)*; and cyclin T, which forms a complex with CDK9 and activates transcription by hyperphosphorylation of the carboxyl-terminal domain of the large subunit of RNA polymerase II *(31)*.

Eleven CDK proteins (Cdc2 = CDK1, CDK2, . . . CDK11) have been discovered and examined in mammalian cells to date. Of these, CDK2, CDK3, CDK4, and CDK6 are principally responsible for G1 progression and entry into S phase. CDK4 and CDK6 are activated in mid G1, whereas CDK2 is activated in late G1. While CDK4 and CDK6 are co-expressed in many cell types, CDK6 does not fully compensate for the function of CDK4 in most cells *(32,33)*. The CDK4/cyclin D and CDK 6/cyclin D complexes play pivotal roles in early to mid G1, whereas CDK2/cyclin E and possibly CDK2/cyclin A function at the late stage of G1 *(22)*. These cyclins are comprehensively termed the G1 cyclins *(34)*. Three types of cyclin Ds (D1, D2, and D3) have been identified, each of which functions as a regulatory subunit of either CDK4 or CDK6 *(35)*. In mid G1 phase, the CDK4/cyclin D complexes phosphorylate the pRB (retinoblastoma) family of nuclear phosphoproteins (*see* **Subheading 2.1.4.**), which are the key regulators of the G1/S transition *(36)*, whereas CDK2/cyclin A and CDK2/cyclin E phosphorylate pRB at the G1 to S transition *(34,37)*.

When quiescent cells enter the cell cycle owing to mitogenic signals, the expression of the cyclin Ds is induced and the CDK4/cyclin D and CDK6/cyclin D complexes are formed as the cells progress through the G1 phase *(38)*. The kinase activity of the complexes is then activated when they enter the cell nucleus and are phosphorylated by CAK. This allows the complexes to phosphorylate target proteins such as pRBs *(39,38)*. Thus, the cyclin D protein types play a pivotal role in G1 by transmitting the mitogenic signal to the pRB/E2F pathway. Notably, cyclin D1 also seems to play a CDK-independent role as a modulator of transcription factors because it interacts with histone acetylases and components of the transcriptional machinery. The cyclin D1–deficient mouse is viable but does have developmental abnormalities that are limited to restricted tissues *(38)*. Proteasomal degradation of cyclin D1 is triggered by its phosphorylation on a single threonine residue (Thr-286) by glycogen synthase kinase-3β *(40)*.

Cyclin E, which regulates CDK2 and possibly also CDK3, is expressed in late G1 and early S phase *(34)*. The level of cyclin E is abruptly decreased by proteolysis after polyubiquitination mediated by SCF (Skp2) ubiquitin ligase *(41)*. Cyclin E regulates the initiation of DNA replication by phosphorylating components of the DNA replication machinery *(39)*. The CDK2/cyclin E complex also triggers the duplication of centrosomes at G1/S phase by phosphorylating the multifunctional protein nucleophosmin (also known as B23) *(42,43)*. CDK2/cyclin E also targets NPAT (nuclear protein mapped to the AT locus) as a phosphorylation substrate, which may explain why CDK activity is linked to the periodic synthesis of histones *(44–46)*.

Cyclin A can activate two different CDKs and functions in both S phase and mitosis *(47)*. Cyclin A starts to accumulate during S phase and is abruptly destroyed before metaphase. The synthesis of cyclin A is mainly controlled at the transcription level and involves E2F and other transcription factors. It is still unknown why CDK2/cyclin A and CDK2/cyclin E complexes are both required for the initiation of DNA replication and why their order of activation is tightly regulated. Using a cell-free system, it has been shown that cyclin E stimulates replication complex assembly by cooperating with Cdc6, a regulator of the initiation of DNA replication, whereas cyclin A has dual functions: first, it activates DNA synthesis by the replication complexes that are already assembled, and second, it inhibits the assembly of new complexes *(48)*. This regulatory mechanism allows cyclin E to promote replication complex assembly while cyclin A blocks this assembly. Thus, the dual functions of cyclin A ensure that the assembly phase (G1) ends before DNA synthesis (S) begins, thereby preventing re-initiation until the next cell cycle.

2.1.2. INK4 Family of CDK Inhibitors

CDK activity is negatively controlled by association with CDK inhibitors (CKIs), which inactivate CDK/cyclin complexes and thereby cause growth arrest *(39,17)*. CKIs are grouped into either the INK4 (inhibitors of CDK4) family or the CIP/KIP family based on their structure and which CDK they target. There are four INK4 CKIs and three CIP/KIP CKIs (*see* **Subheading 2.1.3.**). The first class of inhibitors includes the INK4 proteins, which specifically inhibit CDK4/cyclin D1-associated kinase activity and are therefore specific for early G1 phase *(49)*. Four such proteins have been identified{\}p16^{INK4a}, p15^{INK4b}, p18^{INK4c}, and p19^{INK4d} *(39)*. These INK4 CKIs compete with cyclin D for binding to CDK4 and consequently cause CDK4/cyclin D complexes to dissociate. Note that the major portion of these molecules is composed of four (p16^{INK4a} and p15^{INK4b}) or five (p18^{INK4c} and p19^{INK4d}) tandem ankyrin (ANK) repeats (**Fig. 1**). This 33-residue repeat was first discovered in ANK, a membrane protein of red cells. Later this motif was found in a wide variety of proteins *(50)*. The beta hairpin helix-loop-helix folds formed by the multiple tandem ANK repeats stack in a linear manner to produce an elongated structure that is considered to be involved in macromolecular recognition. p16^{INK4a}, which consists of four ANK repeats (**Fig. 1**), represents the minimal ANK folding unit *(51)*.

Of these CKIs, only the p16^{INK4a} gene (also known as major tumor suppressor 1 or *MTS-1*) has been classified as a tumor suppressor by the genetic criteria of loss of heterozygosity (LOH) *(49)*. Unlike other tumor suppressor genes, *p16* is often silenced by homozygous deletions at the p16^{INK4a} locus (9p21) that also often inactivate two other important genes nearby, namely *p15INK4b* and *p14ARF* (*see* **Subheading 2.3.**).

2.1.3. CIP/KIP Family of CDK Inhibitors

The second family of CDK inhibitors is composed of the more broadly acting CIP/KIP proteins, such as p21$^{CIP1/WAF1}$, p27^{KIP1}, and p57^{KIP2}, which inhibit the activities of cyclin D-, E-, and A-dependent kinases and induce cell cycle arrest *(39)*. Thus, these CKIs are not specific for a particular phase of the cell cycle. Unlike the INK4 proteins, the CIP/KIP proteins associate with the CDK-cyclin complexes and thus do not dissociate these complexes *(39,52)*. The CIP/KIP proteins share a homologous domain at their N-termini that is believed to

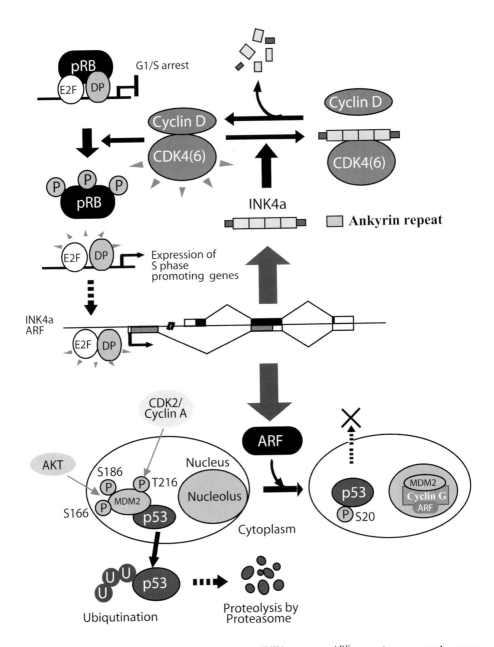

Fig. 1. The *INK4a/ARF* locus encodes p16^{INK4a} and p19^{ARF}, two degenerated tumor suppressor proteins. Absence of p16^{INK4a} (composed of ANK) activates CDK4(6)/ cyclin D kinase, which phosphorylates pRB, thereby activating the E2F/DP1 transcription factor. Since the transcription of the *ARF* gene is regulated by E2F, expression of ARF is induced. ARF separates MDM2 from p53 by recruiting MDM2 into the nucleolus, possibly in collaboration with cyclin G1 and cyclin G2. This stabilizes p53 in the nucleus and allows it to activate the expression of the target genes that function in cell cycle checkpoint, DNA repair, and apoptosis. Thus, the *INK4a/ARF* locus influences both the pRB-E2F and p53 pathways.

participate in the CKI role of these proteins. This amino-terminal domain contains characteristic motifs that are used for binding to both the CDK and cyclin subunits. This association of CIP/KIP proteins with CDK/cyclin complexes has an inhibitory effect. For example, it inhibits CDK2 activity by preventing its Thr-160 phosphorylation by CAK.

p21[WAF1] was discovered almost simultaneously by several studies, each of which employed different approaches. It was discovered as a CDK2-associated protein by a two-hybrid system *(53)*, as a senescent cell-derived inhibitor (Sdi1) of cellular growth *(54)*, as a potential mediator of p53 tumor suppression that was named wild-type p53-activated fragment (WAF1) *(55)*, and as a biochemically isolated CDK2/cyclin-binding protein *(56)*. Transcription of the *p21WAF1* gene can be induced by the tumor suppressor p53 *(55)*, by the antimitogenic cytokine transforming growth factor (TGF)-β *(57)*, and by the phorbol ester tetradecanoyl-phorbol acetate (TPA), which is a protein kinase C activator *(58)*.

Apart from their role as CDK inhibitors, the CIP/KIP proteins may also act to bridge the bond between CDK4 (or CDK6) and cyclin D protein types (but not other CDKs or cyclins), thereby enhancing this association and promoting the recruitment of the CDK/cyclin D complexes to the nucleus *(52,59,60)*. A fact supporting this notion is that mouse fibroblasts that lack both p21[WAF1] and p27[KIP1] are unable to assemble detectable amounts of CDK/cyclin D complexes, and fail to efficiently direct cyclin D proteins into the nucleus *(61)*. These effects were reversed by returning the CKIs to these cells. Thus, unlike the INK4 family proteins, the CIP/KIP CKIs promote the formation of CDK4/cyclin D complexes *(62)*.

In the nucleus, p21[WAF1] binds to proliferating cell nuclear antigen (PCNA) and blocks DNA replication *(63–65)*. p21[WAF1] may also regulate the transcription of the genes involved in growth arrest, senescence, aging, or apoptosis after DNA damage *(52)*.

2.1.4. Retinoblastoma Family of Proteins and E2F

The tumor suppressor pRB is the protein product of the retinoblastoma (Rb) susceptibility gene that is required for the arrest in the G1 phase of the cell cycle *(66,67)*. pRB, and the related p107 and p130 proteins, share structural and functional properties and interact with a number of common cellular targets. Consequently, they form together the "pocket protein family" *(36,68)* **(Fig. 1)**. They function as transcriptional repressors in the nucleus and inhibit the activity of the E2F (early gene 2 factor) transcription factor that regulates the expression of the many genes required for S phase entry and DNA synthesis *(69)*. Although the pRB proteins do not interact directly with DNA, they repress E2F-regulated genes in two ways. First, they directly bind to the transactivation domain of E2F proteins to repress their transcriptional activity.

Second, they recruit chromatin remodeling enzymes such as histone deacetylases (HDACs) or methyl transferases to the nearby surrounding nucleosome structure *(46,70)*.

In the early G1 phase, pRBs are not phosphorylated and can associate with more than eighty proteins, including the E2F family of transcription factors. As G1 progresses, however, the pRB proteins become phosphorylated on multiple serine and threonine residues, primarily by the CDK4/cyclin D or CDK6/cyclin D complexes, but also partly by CDK2/cyclin E *(71)*. This hyperphosphorylation inactivates the pRB proteins and causes them to release their cargo proteins, which activates the cargo proteins and allows them to mediate the events that are required for further cell cycle progression *(39,72)*. The phosphorylation of pRB by the CDK4(6)/cyclin D complexes releases histone deacetylase, which alleviates transcriptional repression, whereas the phosphorylation by CDK2/cyclin E disrupts the pocket domain of pRB, causing the pRB–E2F complex to dissociate *(73)*. Recently, it was suggested that the acetylation of pRB proteins may also influence their activity *(74)*.

The E2F transcription factor was first identified as a transcriptional activity that influences the adenovirus E2 gene promoter *(75)*. The family of E2F-related proteins include E2F1–E2F6. These proteins have conserved DNA-binding and dimerization domains, and three heterodimeric partners, namely DP1, DP2, and DP3 *(76,77)*. Of the six E2Fs, E2F6 is exceptional in that it lacks the domains required for transactivation and pRB binding that are normally in the E2F carboxy-termini. E2F6 appears to play a pRB-independent role in gene silencing and modulation of G0 phase *(78,79)*. Recent studies have expanded the roles that are played by the E2F family of transcription factors. It now appears that apart from being transcriptional regulators of genes involved in DNA metabolism and DNA synthesis, these proteins also seem to play contrasting roles in transcriptional activation and repression, proliferation and apoptosis, tumor suppression and oncogenesis, and possibly differentiation and DNA repair *(66,69,76,80,81)*.

2.1.5. Cdc25A Phosphatase

Cdc25, a dual-specificity phosphatase, removes inhibitory phosphates from the tyrosine and threonine residues of CDKs and thereby promotes cell cycle progression *(82)*. Three Cdc25 homologs, namely Cdc25A, Cdc25B, and Cdc25C, have been identified in mammalian cells. Cdc25C promotes the G2/M transition by activating CDK1 (Cdc2), whereas Cdc25B is proposed to act as a "starter phosphatase" that initiates the positive feedback loop at the entry into M phase *(83,84)*. In contrast, Cdc25A plays an important role in the G1/S transition *(85)*. Overexpression of Cdc25A activates CDK2/cyclin E or CDK2/cyclin A by inducing CDK2 tyrosine dephosphorylation. The activated CDK2/

cyclin complexes then abrogate checkpoint-induced arrest in S phase *(86,104,199)*. Without Cdc25A activity, the inhibitory tyrosine phosphorylation of CDK2 would persist, which would maintain the block of entry into S phase and DNA replication. Cdc25A and Cdc25B (but not Cdc25C) are potential human oncogenes that have been found to be overexpressed in a subset of aggressive human cancers *(87,88)*.

To activate the protein kinase activity of CDK2, it must be phosphorylated on Thr-160 but not on Thr-14 and Tyr-15 *(89)*. A multi-subunit enzyme CAK, which consists of cyclin H and CDK7, phosphorylates CDK2 on Thr-160 *(90,91)*, whereas the KAP phosphatase dephosphorylates Thr-160 in the absence of cyclin, thereby rendering CDK2 inactive *(92)*. CDK2 is phosphorylated on Thr-14 and Tyr-15 by Wee1/Mik1-related protein kinases, whereas the Tyr-15 residue and possibly also the Thr-14 residue are dephosphorylated by Cdc25A *(93)*. Thus, downregulation of Cdc25A leads to growth arrest in late G1 *(94)*. Transcription of the *cdc25A* gene is inhibited by the E2F-4/p130 complex, which recruits histone deacetylase to the E2F site of the *cdc25A* promoter in response to TGF-β *(95)*.

As a cellular response to ultraviolet light (UV)-induced DNA damage, Cdc25A is highly degraded by ubiquitin- and proteasome-dependent proteolysis *(96)*. The same degradation also occurs after hydroxyurea (HU)-triggered stalling of replication forks *(97)* as well as during the midblastula transition in *Xenopus* embryos under physiological conditions *(98)*. Following DNA damage, Cdc25A is phosphorylated by checkpoint kinase 1 (CHK1) or checkpoint kinase 2 (CHK2) (**Fig. 2B**). This phosphorylation is recognized as a tag by the proteolysis system and Cdc25A is degraded. Thus, CHK1 or CHK2 induces the G1/S phase checkpoint by phosphorylating Cdc25A (*see* **Subheading 4.2.**). Supporting this is the finding that the elimination of CHK1 expression through the use of siRNA not only abrogated the S or G2 arrest, it also protected Cdc25A from degradation*(88)*. During the basal turnover in unperturbed S phase, CHK1 phosphorylates serines 75, 123, 178, 278, and 292 of Cdc25A. In contrast, ionizing radiation (IR)-induced Cdc25A proteolysis is mediated by a combined action of CHK1 and CHK2. Thus, a CHK1-CHK2 inhibitor may be useful in cancer chemotherapy, as it may potentiate the cytotoxicity caused not only by DNA-damaging drugs that induce G2 arrest but also by agents that promote S arrest *(99,100)*.

2.1.6. Myc

The c-*myc* protooncogene is a pivotal regulator of cellular proliferation, growth, differentiation, and apoptosis *(101)*. The Myc family proteins (Myc, N-Myc, and L-Myc) are transcription factors with basic helix-loop-helix leucine zipper protein (bHLH-ZIP) motifs that bind to the DNA sequence

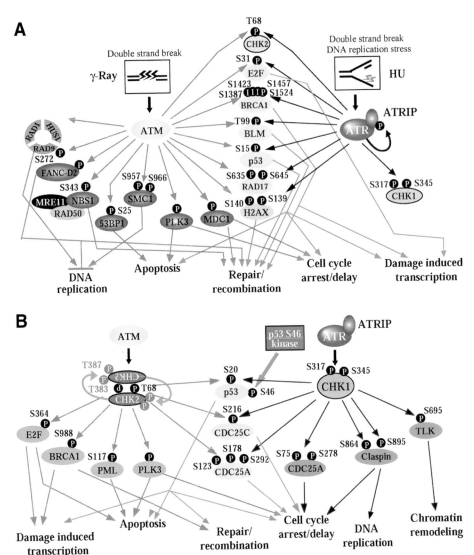

Fig. 2. ATM/ATR and CHK1/CHK2 kinases mediate the signaling network of the DNA damage and DNA replication checkpoints. (**A**) Phosphorylation target proteins of ATM and ATR kinases. There are two parallel pathways that respond to DNA damaging stress in mammalian cells. The ATM pathway responds to the presence of DSBs acting at all phases of the cell cycle. The ATR pathway not only responds to DSBs but also to the agents that disturb the function of replication forks. Following their activation by DSBs or replication stress, ATM/ATR kinases phosphorylate unique (red and black, respectively) or overlapping (green) target proteins at specific serine (S) or threonine (T) residues of indicated (if known) numbers. (**B**) Phosphorylation target

CACGTG (E-box) when dimerized with Max, another bHLH-ZIP. A head-to-tail pair of Myc-Max dimers form a heterotetramer that is capable of bridging distant E-boxes. Mitogen exposure promptly induces the expression of c-*myc*. Ectopic expression of c-*myc* also encourages quiescent cells to enter into S phase *(102)*. Myc not only targets genes that encode cyclins D2, D1 and E, and Cdc25A as a transcription factor, but also sequesters p27^{KIP1} into CDK4(6)/cyclin D complexes away CDK2/cyclin E to cause phosphorylation and subsequent ubiquitination and proteasome-mediated degradation of the p27^{KIP1}, thereby realizing at least three distinct regulatory functions of CDK2/Cyclin E activity, E2F-dependent transcription, and cell growth *(103)*.

In association with Max, Myc binds to the E-boxes in a variety of gene promoters and thus orchestrates the transcriptional activation of a diverse set of genes. However, Myc on its own inhibits the transcription of other genes, including *p21WAF1* *(104)* and another cyclin-dependent kinase inhibitor, *p15INK4b* *(105,106)*. The DNA-binding protein Miz-1 directly recruits Myc to the *p21WAF1* promoter, where Myc selectively inhibits bound p53 from activating *p21WAF1* transcription and favors the initiation of apoptosis *(107)*. Thus, Myc can influence the outcome of a p53 response in favor of cell death.

2.2. The p53-pRB Pathway Controls the G1/S Transition

The *p53* tumor suppressor gene (TP53) is the most frequently mutated gene (about 50%) in human tumors, and encodes a 53 kDa transcription factor (p53) that directly induces the expression of a substantial number of genes that are important for cell cycle regulation, DNA damage repair, and apoptosis *(108,109)*. Of the genes that are induced by p53, p21^{WAF1} plays a pivotal role in G1 arrest by inhibiting CDK4(6)/cyclin D1 activity, thereby reducing the phosphorylation of pRB and promoting G1 arrest of the cell cycle. This interconnecting signaling pathway involving p53, pRB, and E2F plays an essential role in G1/S transition of the cell cycle. p21^{WAF1} is also known to inhibit S phase progression (G1 arrest) by binding to PCNA, a ring protein that promotes DNA replication *(63)*. The expression level of p53 is low in the absence

---

Fig. 2. *(continued)* proteins of CHK1 and CHK2 kinases. CHK2 is primarily phosphorylated by ATM (and partially by ATR), whereas CHK1 is phosphorylated by ATR. Then, CHK1/CHK2 kinases transmit the checkpoint signals by phosphorylating unique (red and black, respectively) or overlapping (green) target proteins at specific serine (S) or threonine (T) residues of indicated numbers. CHK2, phosphorylated on Thr-68 by ATM, is activated to autophosphorylate on Thr-383 and Thr-387 (blue arrows), further enhancing its kinase activity. Ser-46 of p53 is presumed to be phosphorylated by putative p53 S46 kinase. These phosphorylated proteins further propagate the signal to the downstream targets, thereby regulating various cellular events.

of cellular stress. However, various types of stress, including DNA damage, induce p53 expression and cause G1 arrest. In cases where the DNA damage is too severe to be repaired, p53 induces apoptosis as a desperate attempt to protect the organism *(19,110, 111)*. This essential role of p53 as a critical brake on tumor development explains why it is so frequently found in cancer cells *(112,113)*.

Other genes that are upregulated by p53 *(112)* include *cyclin G1 (27)*, *MDM2* (murine double murine 2), *BAX* (bcl2-associated X protein), *GADD45 (114)*, *14-3-3σ (115)*, *CDK4 (116)*, *p53R2 (117,118)*, *p53AIP1 (119)*, *p53DINP1 (120)*, and *p53RDL1 (121)*. Cyclin G1 and MDM2 regulate the stability of the p53 protein (*see* **Subheading 2.3.**). Bax forms a homodimer or heterodimer with Bcl2, and increasing amounts of the Bax homodimer trigger cytochrome-*c* release from mitochondria, thus promoting apoptosis *(122)*. Gadd45 (induced after growth arrest and DNA damage) is involved in regulating nucleotide excision repair of UV-damage together with p53 and another p53-downstream gene, *p48XPE (123)*. The 14-3-3σ protein associates with and recruits Cdc25C from the nucleus to inhibit the activation of CDK1/cyclin B, thus causing G2 arrest. p53R2 is a homolog of ribonucleotide reductase small subunit (R2). Expression of p53R2, but not that of R2, is induced by DNA damage and serves to supply the cell with the deoxyribonucleotides needed for DNA repair. p53RDL1 (p53-regulated receptor for death and life) interacts with its ligand Netrin-1 and promotes the survival of damaged cells against apoptosis.

At least some of the eleven phosphorylation sites identified on p53 seem to play pivotal roles in its regulation. Three functionally important domains have been identified in the p53 molecule, and phosphorylation at these sites is considered to influence the structural changes of these domains. The middle domain constitutes the core domain that associates with the specific nucletotide sequences at the promoter regions of its target genes. This domain harbors the vast majority of the p53 "hot spot" mutations found in human cancers. In cells with damaged DNA, Ser-15 of p53 is phosphorylated by ATM (ataxia telangiectasia mutated) or ATR (ATM-Rad3-related) *(124–126)*. The ATM gene was first isolated from patients with the autosomal recessive disorder ataxia telangiectasia (A-T). These patients exhibit cerebellar degeneration, immunodeficiency, radiation sensitivity, and predisposition to cancer *(127)*. Phosphorylation of p53 at Ser-20 by CHK1 or CHK2 may also be important for regulating the interaction between p53 and MDM2 *(128,129)*. Upon severe DNA damage, Ser-46 on p53 is phosphorylated and apoptosis is induced. As p53AIP1 (p53-regulated apoptosis-inducing protein 1) is selectively induced by p53 molecules that have been phosphorylated at Ser-46, it may be that p53AIP1 mediates this p53-dependent apoptosis by inducing the release of cytochrome-*c* from mitochondria *(130)*. p53DINP1 (p53-dependent damage-inducible nuclear protein 1) functions as a cofactor of the putative p53-Ser46 kinase that promotes phosphorylation of p53 at Ser-46 *(120)*.

2.3. Regulation of p53 Stability by ARF and MDM2

The *INK4a* locus that generates p16^{INK4a} also encodes a degenerated gene product called ARF (after alternative reading frame) *(131)*. Thus, the locus encodes two tumor suppressor proteins, p16^{INK4a} and p19^{ARF} (p14^{ARF} in humans), which activate the growth suppressive functions of pRB and p53, respectively *(67)*. ARF is a highly basic (pI > 12), arginine-rich nucleolar protein *(132)*. Deletion of the *ARF* gene can inactivate p53 function in tumors where p53 itself remains intact. Transcription of the *ARF* gene is regulated by E2F, and thus the *INK4a/ARF* locus influences both the pRB-E2F and p53 pathways.

Overexpression in the same tumor lines of MDM2 (murine double murine 2; Hdm2 in humans), a protein whose expression is upregulated by p53 (*see* **Subheading 2.2.**), has the same effect. This is because ARF binds to MDM2 and abrogates its p53-inhibitory activity. MDM2 destabilizes p53 by catalyzing its ubiquitination by acting as an E3 ubiquitin ligase. This promotes the nuclear export of p53, thereby allowing it to be targeted for proteasomal degradation *(133,134)*. Actually, MDM2 is frequently overexpressed in human tumors, and this leads to the rapid degradation of p53 *(135)*. Since MDM2 directly binds to the N-terminus of p53, phosphorylations of p53 at Ser-15, Ser-20, and Thr-18 are important for the dissociation of MDM2 from p53 *(128,129)*. MDM2 is itself transcriptionally activated by p53, which thus creates a negative feedback loop. Consequently, inhibiting the interaction between p53 and MDM2 by the application of synthetic molecules may serve as an effective cancer treatment because it may lead to cell cycle arrest or apoptosis in p53-positive tumor cells *(109)*.

Other proteins also modulate MDM2 activity. Mitogen-induced activation of phosphatidylinositol 3-kinase (PI3-kinase) and its downstream target, the AKT/PKB serine-threonine kinase, results in the phosphorylation of MDM2 on Ser-166 and Ser-186. CDK2/cyclin A also phosphorylates MDM2 on Thr-216 *(136)*. These phosphorylation events are necessary for the translocation of MDM2 from the cytoplasm into the nucleus and thus serve to promote the p53-inhibitory activity of MDM2 as a ubiquitin ligase *(134)*. Cyclin G1 directly binds to MDM2 *(137)*, recruits PP2A (protein phosphatase 2A) to dephosphorylate MDM2 at Thr-216, and releases MDM2 from p53, thereby cooperating with ARF to restrict the ability of MDM2 to negatively regulate p53 *(138)* (**Fig. 1**). Indeed, cyclin G1$^{-/-}$ mouse embryo fibroblasts show enhanced accumulation of p53 and are partially deficient in an irradiation-induced G2/M-phase checkpoint *(139)*. Cyclin G2 may also have redundant or compensatory functions, because it associates with many of the same proteins to which cyclin G1 binds, including p53, PP2A, MDM2, and ARF *(137)*. This p53-stabilizing effect of PP2A/cyclin G complexes may also influence the malignancy of cancer cells, considering that enhanced expression of a truncated form of PP2A was observed in highly metastatic melanoma cells *(140)*. Cells overexpressed with this truncated form of PP2A show irradiation-induced checkpoint defects and appear to elevate genetic instability, which may promote tumor progression *(141)*. These data suggest that cyclin G1 is a positive feedback regulator of p53, since it downregulates the activity of MDM2, which would otherwise restrain the accumulation of p53 *(142)*.

3. DNA Damage Checkpoints

DNA damage caused by IR, chemical reagents, or similar environmental insults induces cell cycle arrest at G1, S, or G2, thereby preventing the replication of damaged DNA or aberrant mitosis until the damage is properly repaired. The molecular mechanism in mammalian cells that detects the presence of double-strand breaks (DSBs) is not well understood. Research in the budding yeast *Saccharomyces cerevisiae,* however, tells us that a quintet complex composed of RAD24, RFC2, RFC3, RFC4, and RFC5 acts in this organism as a sensor of DSBs *(143)*. Disruption of these components causes defects in the damage checkpoint machinery of *S. cerevisiae (144)*. The same DSB-sensing mechanism is also used in another useful yeast strain, *Schizosaccharomyces pombe (145,146)*. In *S. cerevisiae,* the signal of the DSB abnormality is transmitted to the ring-shaped hetero-trimer that is composed of Ddc1/Rad17/Mec3 (Rad9/Rad1/Hus1 in fission yeast and mammals). This hetero-trimer resembles the replication factor PCNA *(147)*. In fission yeast, this complex activates Rad3 kinase, which then phosphorylates CHK1 *(148)*. The activated CHK1 then targets Cdc25C for phosphorylation. Cdc25C is subsequently recognized by Rad24, a 14-3-3 protein (*see* **Subheading 2.2.**), which recruits it out from the nucleus into the cytoplasm, where it inactivates the CDK1/cyclin B complex (Cdc2/Cdc13 in *S. pombe*), which results in G2/M arrest *(149)*. The 14-3-3 proteins bind to serine/threonine-phosphorylated residues in a specific manner and regulate key proteins involved in various physiological processes such as the cell cycle, intracellular signaling, apoptosis, and transcription regulation *(150)*. Similar checkpoint regulatory mechanisms involving 14-3-3 proteins are also employed in vertebrate cells *(2,86,151)*. For example, human CHK1 is activated by phosphorylation and thereby phosphorylates Cdc25C on Ser-216, which is recognized by the 14-3-3σ protein. The14-3-3σ protein then removes Cdc25C from the nucleus to the cytoplasm, thereby preventing the activation of the CDK1/cyclin B complex and entry into mitosis *(3,152–154)*.

In mammalian cells, there are two parallel pathways that respond to DNA-damaging stresses (**Fig. 2**). The first pathway is the ATM pathway, which responds to the presence of DSBs at all phases of the cell cycle. The second pathway is the ATR (ATM-Rad3-related) pathway, which responds not only to DSBs but also to the agents that interfere with the function of replication forks *(126,4,127)*. A third pathway may involve the newly identified ATX (ATM-related X protein), which phosphorylates and activates CHK1 and/or CHK2 *(126,127,155)*. As shown in **Fig. 2**, ATM phosphorylates many target proteins at their specific serine or threonine residues and activates their functions. In response to IR, for example, ATM phosphorylates RAD9 on Ser-272 *(156)*; PLK3, which further phosphorylates CHK2, contributing to its full activation *(157)*; SMC1 (the cohesin protein) on Ser-957 and Ser-966 *(158,159)*; H2AX on Ser-140, which is required for 53BP1 accumulation at DNA break areas *(160)*; 53BP1 on Ser-6, Ser-25/Ser-29, and Ser-784 *(161)*; and MDC1 *(162)*.

The human ATR protein complexes stably with a protein called ATRIP (ATR-interacting protein). These complexes localize in nuclear foci after damage and thus appear to be recruited to the sites of DNA damage *(163)*. The ATR homologs in fission yeast (Rad3) and budding yeast (Mec1) also form similar complexes with the ATRIP-related factors Rad26 and Ddc2/Lcd2/Pie1, respectively, which are also recruited to the sites of DNA damage *(164–167)*. ATR phosphorylates H2AX on Ser-139 *(168)*, whereas ATM/ATR phosphorylate E2F on Ser-31 *(169)*. The checkpoint functions of ATM in response to IR are primarily mediated by the effector kinase CHK2, whereas those of ATR in response to replication inhibition and UV-induced damage are mediated by CHK1. Thus, the structurally unrelated CHK2 and CHK1 proteins channel the DNA damage signals from ATM and ATR, respectively *(21,170)*. However, recent observations suggest the existence of various "crosstalks" among these kinases *(100,171)*, and the presence of a novel checkpoint cascade signaling by way of ATM-CHK1 to Tousled-like kinases (TLKs) that causes chromatin remodeling in response to various stresses *(172)*.

The expression of the labile CHK1 protein is restricted to the S and G2 phases *(173)*. Although it is active even in unperturbed cell cycles, it is further activated in response to DNA damage or stalled replication *(100,174)*. Following a checkpoint signal, CHK1 is phosphorylated on Ser-317 and Ser-345 by ATR in cooperation with the sensor complexes, which include the mammalian homologs of Rad17 and Hus1. The phosphorylation at the Ser-345 site is required for nuclear retention of CHK1 following an HU-induced checkpoint signal *(175–177)*. CHK1 not only stimulates the kinase activity of DNA-dependent protein kinase (DNA-PK) complexes, which leads to increased phosphorylation of p53 on Ser-15 and Ser-37; it also elevates the DNA-PK-dependent end-joining reactions, thereby promoting the repair of DSBs *(178)*. *CHK1⁻/⁻* mice show a severe proliferation defect and death in embryonic stem (ES) cells and peri-implantation embryonic lethality. The ES cells lacking CHK1 have also been shown to have a defective G2/M DNA damage checkpoint in response to IR *(179,180)*. In contrast, CHK1-deficient cells called DT40 are viable, but they fail to arrest at G2/M in response to IR and fail to maintain viable replication forks when DNA polymerase is inhibited *(181)*.

In contrast, the other Ser/Thr protein CHK2 kinase (also known as hCds1) must be phosphorylated at Thr-68 by ATM to activate it in response to IR-induced DNA damage (this is not the case for damage owing to UV or HU) *(170,182)*. Unlike CHK1, CHK2 is a stable protein that is expressed throughout the cell cycle and that seems to be inactive in the absence of DNA damage *(173)*. Its activation involves its dimerization and autophosphorylation. Unlike the catalytically inactive form of CHK2, wild-type CHK2 leads to G1 arrest after DNA damage by phosphorylating p53 on Ser-20, which causes the pre-formed p53/MDM2 complexes to dissociate and increases the stability of p53 *(128)*. Unlike *ATM⁻/⁻* and *p53⁻/⁻* mice, *CHK2⁻/⁻* mice do not spontaneously develop tumors, although the IR-induced G1/S cell cycle checkpoint—but not the G2/M or S phase checkpoints—was impaired in primary mouse embryonic fibroblasts (MEFs) derived from *CHK2⁻/⁻* mice *(183,184)*.

That the fission yeast homolog of CHK2, Cds1, may participate in repair is suggested by the finding that it interacts with the Mus81–Eme1 endonuclease complex, which can resolve the Holliday junction *(185,186)*. The human Mus81–Eme1 complex also has a similar function as a flap/fork endonuclease that is likely to play a role in the processing of stalled replication fork intermediates *(187)*.

CHK1 and CHK2 share partly redundant roles in that they target common downstream effector proteins such as the Polo-like kinase 3 (PLK3) *(188)*, the promyelocytic leukemia (PML) protein *(189)*, the E2F1 transcription factor *(190)*, or the TLKs *(172)*. PLK3 binds to and phosphorylates p53 on Ser-20. Through this direct regulation of p53 activity, PLK3 is at least partly involved in regulating the DNA damage checkpoint as well as M-phase function. The *PML* gene is translocated in most acute promyelocytic leukemias and encodes a tumor suppressor protein that plays a pivotal role in gamma irradiation–induced apoptosis. It is proposed that CHK2 mediates gamma irradiation–induced apoptosis in a p53-independent manner through an ATM-CHK2-PML pathway *(189)*. PML also recruits CHK2 and p53 into the PML-nuclear bodies, and enhances the p53/CHK2 interaction to protect p53 from MDM2-mediated ubiquitination and degradation *(191)*. Mutations in the prototypic member of the Tousled (Tsl) kinase from the plant *Arabidopsis thaliana* lead to a pleiotropic phenotype *(192)*. In mammals, however, the TLKs are regulated in a cell cycle-dependent manner that peaks at S phase and are involved in chromatin assembly by phosphorylating the chromatin assembly factors Asf1a and Asf1b *(193)*. CHK1 phosphorylates TLK1 on Ser-695 in vitro, and substitution of Ser-695 with alanine impairs the efficient downregulation of TLK1 after DNA damage *(172)*.

4. G1 Checkpoint Response

In mid-to-late G1, and if the cellular environment is favorable for proliferation, a binary decision—whether to commit to the mitotic cell cycle and enter S-phase, or whether to not commit to the cell cycle and remain in a quiescent, non-proliferative state—is made at the "restriction point" *(194,195)*. As described above, many proteins are involved in making this critical decision and in ensuring proper progression of the G1/S transition. Although cyclin D meets the criteria of the critical restriction point factor, the system seems to be far more complex than just relying on a single factor. Moreover, the relationship between the restriction point and DNA damage checkpoints remains elusive *(196)*. The cell cycle checkpoints that monitor the proper G1/S transition and S phase progression during potentially hazardous genotoxic stress *(103, 197)* will be discussed in the following sections.

4.1. The ATM(ATR)/p53-Mediated Pathway

The ATM(ATR)/p53 pathway plays a pivotal role in one of the checkpoint mechanisms that arrest the cell cycle at G1 phase following DNA damage (G1 checkpoint) **(Fig. 3)**. As described in **Subheading 3,** ATM is activated in response to IR, whereas ATR is activated in response to replication inhibition or UV-induced damage. The activated ATM or ATR then phosphorylates p53 (on Ser-15), and this phosphorylation causes MDM2 to dissociate from p53, which stabilizes p53 and leads to its accumulation *(128,129)*. Increased expression of ARF owing to E2F1 stabilization in response to DNA damage also blocks the inhibitory function of MDM2, thereby increasing the nuclear amount of p53.

The principal kinases relaying ATM(ATR)-initiated checkpoint signaling are preferentially CHK2 for ATM and CHK1 for ATR. In response to IR or DNA replication stress, ATR phosphorylates CHK1 at Ser-317 and Ser-345 *(175,177,198)*, which moderately increases its kinase activity and allows it to propagate the signal to downstream effectors, including p53, which CHK1 phosphorylates on Ser-20 *(129)*. In response to IR, ATM phosphorylates CHK2 at Thr-68 *(199)*, followed by CHK2 autophosphorylation on Thr-383 and Thr-387 and the activation of several target proteins, including p53, which CHK2 also phosphorylates on Ser-20 *(128,129)*. These Ser-20 phosphorylation events both induce MDM2 to dissociate from p53.

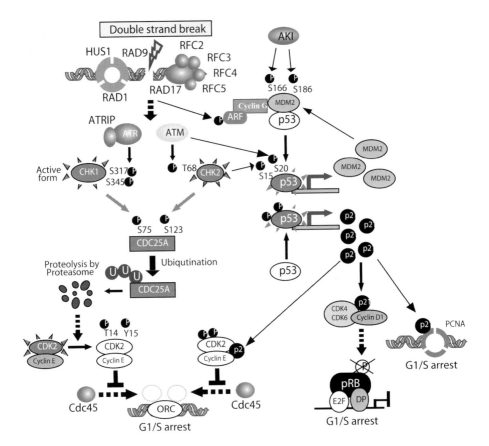

Fig. 3. ATM(ATR)-mediated G1/S checkpoint pathways. DNA damage triggers a rapid cascade of phosphorylation events involving either the ATM and CHK2 (upon IR) or the ATR and CHK1 (upon UV light) kinases. These phosphorylation events activate the target protein kinases to trap and phosphorylate the next target proteins, thereby transmitting the DNA damage signals. It has been determined that in response to IR, ATM phosphorylates CHK2 at Thr-68, whereas ATR (or ATM) phosphorylates CHK1 at Ser-317 and Ser-345. In one pathway (left), the CHK2 or CHK1 kinase phosphorylates Cdc25A phosphatase at serines 75, 123, 178, 278, and 292 (100). Of these, the Ser-123 residue that is targeted by CHK2 and the Ser-75 residue that is phosphorylated by CHK1 seem to be particularly critical residues of Cdc25A (202, 99). The phosphorylated Ser-123 or Ser-75 residue is recognized by the ubiquitination (Ub) enzyme, and this promotes the rapid degradation of Cdc25A by the proteasome. Due to the disappearance of Cdc25A phosphatase activity that this degradation causes, the CDK2/cyclin E complex is locked in its inactive form because of the presence of the inhibitory phosphorylation on the Thr-14 and Tyr-15 residues of CDK2. Thus, the CDK2/cyclin E complex fails to load Cdc45 onto chromatin and the blockade of the initiation of the DNA replication origins is maintained.

The stabilized and activated p53 protein that results from CHK1/CHK2-mediated phosphorylation induces the transcription of a large number of genes, including *p21*^{WAF1}, which silences the kinase activities of the CDK2/cyclin E, CDK2/cyclin A, or CDK4(6)/cyclin D complexes. This prevents the complexes from loading the Cdc45 origin binding factor onto chromatin, which precludes the recruitment of DNA polymerases, thereby blocking initiation of DNA replication from the unfired origins *(200,201)*. Another important consequence of inhibiting both the CDK2 and CDK4(6) kinase complexes is that these complexes cannot then phosphorylate pRB, which allows pRB to maintain its inhibition of the E2F-dependent transcription of S-phase genes that are essential for S-phase entry as described in **Subheading 2.1.4.** These effects all result in G1 arrest. Maintenance of the G1/S arrest by way of this pathway after DNA damage is a delayed response that requires the transcription, translation, and/or protein stabilization of key checkpoint transducers. However, once initiated, this pathway provides a long-lasting G1 arrest, and the entry into S phase is prevented as long as a single unrepaired DNA lesion is detected by the checkpoint machinery.

4.2. The ATR(ATM)/Cdc25A-Mediated Pathway

The human Cdc25A phosphatase plays a pivotal role at the G1/S transition because it enhances the kinase activities of the CDK2/cyclin E and CDK2/cyclin A complexes by dephosphorylating the inhibitory phosphorylated Thr-14 and Tyr-15 residues of CDK2 *(102197)*. After UV and IR exposure, Cdc25A is ubiquinated because it is phosphorylated by CHK1 (in the case of UV)

Fig. 3. *(continued)* In the other pathway (right), Ser-15 of p53 is directly phosphorylated by ATM or ATR in cells with damaged DNA. The phosphorylation of p53 at Ser-20 by CHK1 or CHK2 induces the dissociation of the p53/MDM2 complex, which increases the stability of p53 because MDM2 primes p53 for ubiquitination and proteasomal degradation (*see* **Fig. 1**). CHK1 also stimulates the kinase activity of DNA-PK complexes, which increases the phosphorylation of p53 on Ser-15 and Ser-37. Furthermore, DNA damage can also upregulate ARF, which specifically inhibits MDM2, putatively in collaboration with the cyclin G proteins. The collective result is that stable and transcriptionally active p53 transcription factor accumulates in the cell nucleus and induces the expression of a large number of target genes, including the p21 CDK inhibitor. The increased p21 levels inhibit the CDK2/cyclin E complex or the CDK4(6)/cyclin D complexes, thus arresting the cell cycle at G1/S phase. Upon severe DNA damage, Ser-46 on p53 is phosphorylated by the putative p53-Ser46 kinase with the aid of p53DINP1, which selectively induces the expression of p53AIP1, which is a mediator of apoptosis because it induces the release of cytochrome-*c* from mitochondria.

(87,96,) and CHK2 (in the case of IR) *(202)*. The critical residue of Cdc25A that is targeted by CHK2 is Ser-123 *(202)*. Cdc25A is also phosphorylated on Ser-75 by CHK1 *(109)*. The phosphorylated Ser-123 residue (and possibly also the phosphorylated Ser-75 residue) is recognized by the ubiquitination (Ub) enzyme, which promotes the rapid degradation of Cdc25A by the proteasome system. Removal of Cdc25A in turn keeps the CDK2-associated kinase complexes in their inactive form due to the persisting inhibitory phosphorylation of their Thr-14 and Tyr-15 residues. This results in G1 arrest. The important target of this cascade is the inhibition of CDK2-dependent loading of Cdc45 onto DNA pre-replication complexes. Thus, the ATM(ATR)–CHK2(CHK1)–Cdc25A–CDK2 pathway accounts for the rapid and p53-independent initiation of the G1 checkpoint, where the abundance and activity of Cdc25A decreases without delay in response to IR- or UV-mediated DNA damage **(Fig. 3)** . It is likely that this regulatory mechanism is conserved among vertebrates and operates in every cell type.

During interphase, CDK2 appears to phosphorylate Cdc25A, which constitutes a Cdc25A-CDK2 autoamplification feedback loop *(203)*. Cdc25A also seems to be involved in the G2/M transition, besides its commonly accepted effect on G1/S progression *(87)*. Proteolysis of Cdc25A is also linked with the intra-S-phase checkpoint, which guards against premature entry into mitosis in the presence of stalled replication forks.

4.3. Other Potential G1 Checkpoint Pathways

It has been reported that there is another G1 checkpoint induced by IR exposure, which is characterized by enhanced protein degradation *(204)*. In this checkpoint, DNA damage unmasks a cryptic "destruction box" (RxxL) within the cyclin D1 amino-terminus that is then recognized by the anaphase-promoting complex (APC) ubiquitin ligase, which primes cyclin D1 for rapid proteasomal destruction *(197)*. This causes the p21[WAF1] protein, which served as an assembly factor of the CDK4(6)/cyclin D1 complexes, to be released. p21[WAF1] is then free to bind to another of its targets, the CDK2/cyclin E complex. This binding inactivates the kinase activity of the complex **(Fig. 3)** . Since the proliferation of many mammalian somatic cells depends on the presence of abundant CDK4(6)/cyclin D1 complexes, the destruction of cyclin D1 together with the inactivation of the S-phase-promoting CDK2/cyclin E strongly induces G1 arrest.

Exposure of epithelial cells to UV light can also lead to yet another G1 checkpoint mechanism. This mechanism involves the gradual accumulation of p16[INK4a], which selectively disrupts the CDK4(6)/cyclin D1 complexes. This again causes the release of p21[WAF1], which can then bind to and inhibit CDK2/cyclin E, thereby resulting in G1 arrest. If these mechanisms are confirmed as cell cycle checkpoints, they would each serve as examples of an ATM-independent, cell-type-restricted response. Note that because cyclins D2 and D3 are not degraded upon DNA damage, these pathways would have little effect in cell types that express several D-type cyclins or lack cyclin D1.

To ensure the exact duplication of the genome during every cell division, which is a basic requirement of every proliferating cell, eukaryotes adopt a strategy that temporally separates the assembly of the pre-replication complex (pre-RC) from the initiation of DNA synthesis **(Fig. 4)** *(201,205)*. A key component of the pre-RC is the hexameric minichromosome maintenance (MCM) protein complex, which consists of the six Mcm2–Mcm7 proteins *(206)*. The MCM complex is presumed to be a helicase functioning in the growing forks, and like other helicase proteins *(207)*, it actually adopts a toroidal structure when observed under a microscope *(208)*. The MCM complex is recruited to the replication origins, where the two protein kinase complexes Cdc7–Dbf4 (in budding yeast) and CDK2/cyclin E trigger a chain reaction that results in the phosphorylation and activation of the MCM complex and finally in the initiation of DNA synthesis *(201,209)*. At the onset of S phase, S-phase kinases promote the association of Cdc45 with MCM at the origins. Upon the formation of the MCM–Cdc45 complex at the origins, the duplex DNA is unwound and various replication proteins, including DNA polymerases, are recruited onto the unwound DNA *(200)*. A "licensing checkpoint" that prevents passage into S phase in the absence of sufficient origin licensing may also exist in mammalian cells *(210)*.

5. The S-Phase Checkpoint

Proliferating cells are always exposed to life-threatening insults that disturb the proper replication and segregation of their genomes into daughter cells. In response to these genotoxic insults, eukaryotic cells have evolved checkpoint mechanisms that monitor the progression of DNA replication at S phase and halt replication if an abnormality is observed **(Fig. 4)**. At least two distinct S-phase checkpoints seem to exist. One of these occurs in response to DNA-replication stress that interferes with the proper progression of the replication forks. The other is an intra-S-phase checkpoint that functions in response to DSBs *(2,4)*. The S-phase checkpoint may also have a function during an unperturbed S phase, because even in the absence of exogenous agents, mutants of the many genes that are involved in this checkpoint show aberrant checkpoint signaling, and some mutants also cause checkpoint induction *(2)*.

5.1. S-Phase Checkpoint in Response to DNA Replication Stress

Several types of agents are known to interfere with the function of replication forks and to elicit the S-phase checkpoint. These include agents that

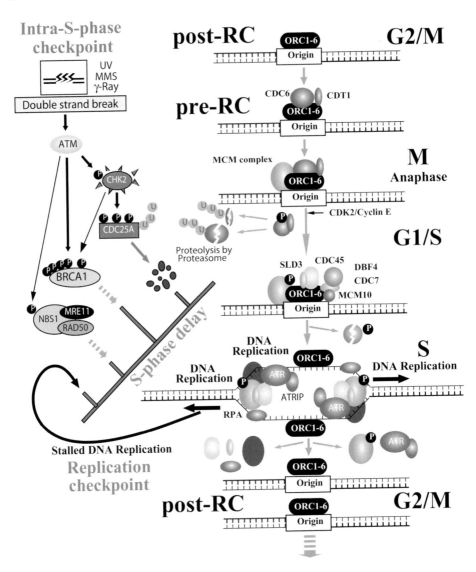

Fig. 4. Molecular mechanism of S-phase progression and the S-phase checkpoints. Upon initiation of DNA replication, DNA replication initiation factors such as MCM10, CDC45–Sld3 (budding yeast) and RPA and checkpoint complexes bind to the pre-replicative complex (pre-RC) on chromatin and trigger the unwinding of DNA. The hexameric MCM2-7 complex is recruited to the replication origins by a number of proteins, including MCM10, RPA, and CDC45–Sld3. The MCM complex is a putative helicase of the growing forks. Two protein kinase complexes, Cdc7/Dbf4 (budding yeast) and CDK2/cyclin E, trigger a chain reaction that results in the phosphorylation of the Mcm complex and finally the initiation of DNA synthesis. The

directly inhibit DNA synthesis. For example, HU stalls replication forks by depleting the deoxynucleotide triphosphate (dNTP) pool, while aphidicolin activates the checkpoint by inhibiting DNA synthesis by blocking the activities of polymerases **(Fig. 4)**. In addition, DNA-modifying agents that block replication can elicit the S-phase checkpoint. These agents include methyl methanesulfonate (MMS) and UV-induced DNA lesions, which slow down the rate of DNA-replication-fork progression in budding yeast *(211)*.

The study of the DNA-replication checkpoint is most advanced in yeasts. However, the checkpoint mechanisms that were unveiled in yeasts also seem to be conserved in mammalian cells *(2,149)*. The central checkpoint kinases Mec1 (ATR in humans) and Rad53 (CHK2 in humans) play an essential role in maintaining DNA replication fork stability in response to DNA damage and replication fork blockage, and they inhibit the activation of late-firing replication origins after HU and MMS exposure *(4)*. The DNA replication forks appear to function both as the activator and as the primary effector of the S-phase checkpoint pathway, since the recruitment of Ddc2 (ATRIP in humans) to nuclear foci and the subsequent activation of the Rad53 kinase occurs only during S phase and requires the assembly of the replication forks *(212)*.

In budding yeast, proteins that are essential for DNA replication, such as DNA polymerase ε and its interacting partners Dpb11 and Drc1/Sld2, are also required for efficient checkpoint activation *(213)*. Dpb11 and its human homolog TopBP1 associate with the PCNA-like protein Ddc1 and human Rad9,

---

Fig. 4. *(continued)* ATR/ATRIP (Rad3/Rad26) complex and the Polα–primase complex and several other replication proteins are also recruited to the unwound DNA. After this, the RAD1/RAD9/HUS1 complex binds to chromatin, an event that requires the RAD17/RFC2-5 complex.

Two kinds of S-phase checkpoint mechanisms are known. One monitors the stalled replication forks (DNA-replication checkpoint) while the other monitors the replication block induced by DSBs during S phase (intra-S-phase checkpoint). In contrast to the checkpoints at the G1/S and G2/M transitions that arrest the cell cycle, these S phase checkpoints can only delay the progression of S phase. Proteins involved in the regulation of DNA replication such as DNA polymerase ε, Dpb11 (TopBP1 in humans), Drc1/Sld2 (budding yeast), Ddc1 (budding yeast), and RPA are also required for the S-phase checkpoint in response to replication blockage. Claspin (Mrc1 in yeast) that is phosphorylated at Ser-864 and Ser-895 by CHK1 also regulates the S-phase checkpoint. ATM is the master transducer of the S-phase checkpoint and phosphorylates BRCA1 and BRCA2 as well as NBS1 (at Ser-343), which is a component of the NBS1/MRE11/RAD50 complex. CHK1 also phosphorylates TLK (at Ser-695), a protein kinase that is potentially involved in regulation of chromatin assembly. Acetylation of nucleosomal histone H3 or H4, which regulates the chromatin structure, and gene expression also play a role in the S-phase checkpoint.

respectively, and seem to collaborate in monitoring the progression of replication forks *(214,215)*. The Polα–primase complex and RPA (replication protein A) are also required for the S-phase checkpoint in response to replication blocks *(216)*.

Claspin, a CHK1-interacting protein, is required for the ATR-dependent activation of CHK1 in *Xenopus* egg extracts that contain incompletely replicated DNA *(217)*. Claspin, ATR, and Rad17 bind to chromatin independently and appear to collaborate in checkpoint regulation by detecting different aspects of the DNA replication fork *(218)*. *Xenopus* Claspin may be phosphorylated at Ser-864 and Ser-895 by CHK1 *(219)*. Human Claspin is a cell cycle-regulated nuclear protein whose levels peak at S/G2 phase and that is phosphorylated in response to replication stress or other types of DNA damage. It appears to work as an adaptor molecule that brings the ATR/CHK1 and RAD9/RAD1/HUS1 complexes together to regulate the S-phase checkpoint *(220)*. These observations suggest that the activation of CHK1 by ATR may be regulated by Claspin in a similar way in budding yeast: Rad9 is phosphorylated by Mec1 in response to DNA damage and subsequently serves as a scaffold protein for Rad53, thus allowing Rad53 to autophosphorylate and self-activate *(221)*. Mrc1, a yeast homolog of Claspin, is also important for the activation of Rad53 and Cds1 in response to HU, and thus may mediate the checkpoint response to replication blockage in a similar manner to Claspin *(222,223)*.

In budding yeast, the S-phase checkpoint activates the ATM-like Mec1 and the CHK2-related Rad53 kinases in response to stalled replication forks that arise owing to replication stress or DNA damage in S phase. These kinases in turn inhibit spindle elongation and late origin firing, which stabilize the DNA polymerases at the arrested forks *(4)*. Orc 2 (origin recognition complex 2) plays a pivotal role in maintaining the number of functional replication forks, and the amount of DNA damage required for Rad53 activation is higher in S phase than in G2 *(224)*. For the S-phase checkpoint, acetylation of the nucleosomal histone H3 or H4 that regulates chromatin structure and gene expression also appears to be important *(225)*. Studies in fission yeast suggest that the signal activating the S-phase checkpoint is generated only when replication forks encounter DNA damage *(226)*.

5.2. S-Phase Checkpoint in Response to DSBs

After DNA damage, proliferating cells actively slow down their DNA replication by activating a checkpoint. This gives the cell time to repair the damage. This checkpoint is often called the intra-S-phase checkpoint (**Fig. 4**) *(4,21)*. The intra-S-phase checkpoint consists of regulatory networks that sense DNA damage and coordinate DNA replication, cell cycle arrest, and DNA repair.

The above-mentioned Cdc25A degradation pathway also appears to induce the transient intra-S-phase response. Here, IR-induced formation of DSBs triggers degradation of Cdc25A, which in turn inhibits the S-phase promoting activity of CDK2/cyclin E and induces the transient blockade of DNA replication, which delays S-phase progression for several hours *(227)*. As described above, Cdc25A destruction involves the phosphorylation of Cdc25A on Ser-123 by both CHK1 and CHK2 in response to IR, and on Ser-75 by CHK1 in response to UV irradiation *(99)*. Supporting the involvement in the S-phase checkpoint of ATM, its phosphorylation targets including CHK2, and the CHK2-regulated Cdc25A-CDK2 cascade, is the fact that mutants of ATM, CDK2, or the other proteins in the CHK2-regulated Cdc25A-CDK2 cascade fail to inhibit S-phase progression when they are irradiated. Consequently, these cells undergo radio-resistant DNA synthesis (RDS), which is a phenomenon of persistent DNA synthesis after irradiation *(127,199)*.

Another phosphorylation target of ATM, the master transducer of the S-phase checkpoint, plays a key role in the intra-S-phase checkpoint, namely, BRCA1 (breast cancer susceptibility gene 1). BRCA2 may also be an important target of ATM *(228,229)*. Mutations in the *BRCA1* and *BRCA2* tumor suppressor genes are responsible for the great majority of familial breast and ovarian cancers. These proteins form nuclear foci with Rad51 during S phase and after DNA damage *(230)*. *BRCA1*- and *BRCA2*-mutant cells exhibit defects in the homologous repair of chromosomal DSBs. *BRCA1* or *BRCA2* deficiency in mice results in early embryonic lethality, but conditional deletions reveal that mice with *BRCA1* or *BRCA2* mutations suffer a wide range of carcinomas *(231)*. Moreover, a mammary epithelium whose *BRCA1* or *BRCA2* gene has been deleted is highly susceptible to mammary tumorigenesis *(232)*. *BRCA1* is omnipresent and plays broad roles in transcriptional regulation that include both p53-dependent and -independent responses. It also has ubiquitin ligase activity when dimerized to Bard1, and undergoes damage-associated phosphorylation by multiple kinases that precedes repair-complex formation *(230)*. In contrast, *BRCA2* has a more straightforward function{\}it is central to homology-directed repair (HDR) because of its interaction with Rad51 and its direct binding to single-stranded DNA *(233)*.

Another important phosphorylation target of ATM that plays a role in the intra-S-phase checkpoint is NBS1 (Nijmegen breakage syndrome gene 1) *(234–236)*. NBS 1 (Xrs2 in yeast) forms a multimeric complex with the MRE11/RAD50 nuclease, MDC1 (mediator of DNA damage checkpoint protein 1), and other unidentified proteins, and recruits them to the vicinity of DNA damage sites by direct binding to the phosphorylated histone H2AX *(237)*. ATM phosphorylates NBS1 at Ser-343 in response to IR *(238)*. Cells harboring a point mutation of NBS1 at this phosphorylation site failed to engage in the S-phase checkpoint induced by IR *(239)*. Moreover, in collaboration with the BRCA1 C-terminus domain, the highly conserved NBS1 forkhead-associated domain plays a crucial role in the recognition of damaged sites *(240)*. After recognizing the DNA damage, the NBS1 complex proceeds to rejoin the DSBs predominantly by homologous recombination repair in vertebrates. This process collaborates with the cell cycle checkpoints at S and G2 phase to facilitate DNA repair.

Mutations in the MRE11-complex genes result in sensitivity to DNA damage, genomic instability, telomere shortening, aberrant meiosis, and abnormal checkpoint signaling in S phase. Blockade of NBS1-MRE11 function and the CHK2-Cdc25A-CDK2 pathway entirely abolishes the inhibition of DNA synthesis that is normally induced by IR. This results in the complete RDS that is also seen when cells harbor a defective ATM gene *(227)*. However, the phosphorylation of NBS1 and CHK2 by ATM seems to trigger two distinct branches of the intra-S-phase checkpoint because CDK2-dependent loading of Cdc45 onto replication origins, a prerequisite for the recruitment of DNA polymerase, is prevented in normal or NBS1/MRE11-defective cells when they are irradiated but not in irradiated cells that harbor a defective ATM protein *(227)*. 53BP1, which plays a partially redundant role in the phosphorylation of the downstream checkpoint effector proteins BRCA1 and CHK2, is also a key transducer of the intra-S-phase and G2-M checkpoint arrests that occur in response to IR *(241)*.

CHK1 may also be necessary for the intra-S-phase checkpoint when DNA synthesis is inhibited by DNA damage *(242)*. Supporting this is that chemical or genetic ablation of human CHK1 triggers the accumulation of Cdc25A, prevents the IR-induced degradation of Cdc25A, and causes RDS *(87)*. Moreover, the basal turnover of Cdc25A operating in unperturbed S phase requires CHK1-dependent phosphorylation of its Ser-123, Ser-178, Ser-278, and Ser-292 residues *(100)*. The ATR-CHK1 pathway may also play an important role in the intra-S-phase checkpoint that is induced by replication-associated DSBs caused by application of the topoisomerase I inhibitor topotecan (TPT) *(243)*, although it has no relationship with DNA-PK activity *(244)*. However, in budding yeast, the intra-S-phase checkpoint control is not activated by another topoisomerase I inhibitor, camptothecin (CPT), and the CPT-hypersensitive mutant strain that fails histone 2A (H2A) Ser-129 phosphorylation is an essential component for the efficient repair of DSBs that do not induce the intra-S-phase checkpoint *(245)*. In *Xenopus* egg extracts, DNA lesions generated by exonuclease or etoposide, a DNA topoisomerase II inhibitor, activate a DNA damage checkpoint that blocks the initiation of DNA replication *(246)*. TLK, a protein kinase that is potentially involved in regulating chromatin assembly and that is phosphorylated by CHK1 on its Ser-695 residue, also appears to be involved in the ATM/CHK1-dependent intra-S-phase checkpoint *(172)*.

Besides its function with H2AX (a histone H2A variant), Mdc1 (mediator of DNA damage checkpoint protein 1) controls damage-induced checkpoints by promoting the recruitment of repair proteins to the sites of DNA breaks *(247)*. Cells that lack the *MDC1* gene are sensitive to IR because they fail to activate the intra-S-phase and G2/M checkpoints properly, probably due to an inability to regulate CHK1 properly. Thus, MDC1 facilitates the establishment of the intra-S-phase cell cycle checkpoint *(248)*. Notably, MDC1 is hyperphosphorylated in an ATM-dependent manner, and rapidly relocalizes to nuclear foci at sites of DNA damage, which appears to be crucial for the efficient activation of the intra-S-phase checkpoint *(249)*.

The ATR/ATRIP complex requires the RFC (replication factor C) and PCNA-like proteins to fully activate the replication-stress response because RFC recognizes the primer-template junction and recruits PCNA onto DNA to function as a sliding clamp that tethers DNA polymerases *(4,250)*. In fission yeast and humans, the PCNA-like complex (Rad1/Rad9/Hus1 or RAD1/RAD9/HUS1) is recruited in a RAD17-dependent manner onto the chromatin after damage *(149,251)*. In budding yeast, the homologous PCNA-like complex (Rad17/Mec3/Ddc1) is recruited to DSBs and the sites of DNA damage in a Rad24-dependent manner *(252,253)*. Thus, it is possible that the Rad17 complex recognizes DNA damage and loads the PCNA-like complex onto DNA, thereby responding to DNA damage independently of ATR/ATRIP *(254)*.

As with fission yeast, RAD17 and HUS1 are required for the phosphorylation of CHK1 by ATR in mammals *(254,255)*. ATR also phosphorylates Rad17 at its Ser-635 and Ser-645 residues *(256)*. This phosphorylation is significantly stimulated by the increased amounts of PCNA-like complexes that were recruited onto the chromatin after damage. Unlike the *hus1*-null fission yeast cells, which are defective for the G2/M DNA-damage checkpoint, mouse cells that lack the mouse homolog of the fission yeast protein Hus1 enter mitosis normally after DNA damage but display an S-phase checkpoint defect *(257)*. The mouse Hus1 protein also seems to play a role in the NBS1-independent checkpoint-mediated inhibition of DNA synthesis that is generated by the genotoxin benzo(a)pyrene dihydrodiol epoxide (BPDE), which causes bulky DNA adducts. However, the *hus1*-null mouse cells displayed intact S-phase checkpoint responses in response to IR-induced DSBs *(257)*.

6. Defects in G1/S Checkpoint and Cancer

Defects in the genome maintenance mechanisms, including DNA repair and cell cycle checkpoint pathways, are believed to enhance genetic instability and

128. Chehab, N. H., Malikzay, A., Appel, M., and Halazonetis, T. D. (2000) Chk2/ hCds1 functions as a DNA damage checkpoint in G(1) by stabilizing p53. *Genes Dev.* **14**, 278–288.

129. Shieh, S. Y., Ahn, J., Tamai, K., Taya, Y., and Prives, C. (2000) The human homologs of checkpoint kinases Chk1 and Cds1 (Chk2) phosphorylate p53 at multiple DNA damage-inducible sites. *Genes Dev.* **14**, 289–300. Erratum in: *Genes Dev.* **14**, 750.

130. Matsuda, K., Yoshida, K., Taya, Y., Nakamura, K., Nakamura, Y., and Arakawa, H. (2002) p53AIP1 regulates the mitochondrial apoptotic pathway. *Cancer Res.* **62**, 2883–2889.

131. Kamijo, T., Zindy, F., Roussel, M. F., Quelle, D. E., Downing, J. R., Ashmun, R. A., et al. (1997) Tumor suppression at the mouse INK4a locus mediated by the alternative reading frame product p19ARF. *Cell* **91**, 649–659.

132. Weber, J. D., Taylor, L. J., Roussel, M. F., Sherr, C. J., and Bar-Sagi, D. (1999) Nucleolar Arf sequesters Mdm2 and activates p53. *Nat. Cell Biol.* **1**, 20–26.

133. Juven-Gershon, T. and Oren, M. (1999) Mdm2: the ups and downs. *Mol. Med.* **5**, 71–83.

134. Mayo, L. D. and Donner, D. B. (2002) The PTEN, Mdm2, p53 tumor suppressor–oncoprotein network. *Trends Biochem. Sci.* **27**, 462–467.

135. Chene, P. (2003) Inhibiting the p53-MDM2 interaction: an important target for cancer therapy. *Nat. Rev. Cancer* **3**, 102–109.

136. Zhang, T. and Prives, C. (2001) Cyclin a-cdk phosphorylation regulates mdm2 protein interactions. *J. Biol. Chem.* **276**, 29702–29710.

137. Kimura, S.H. and Nojima, H. (2002) Cyclin G1 mediates the association of MDM2 with ARF and promotes p53 accumulation. *Genes Cells* **7**, 869–880.

138. Okamoto, K., Li, H. Y., Jensen, M. R., Zhang, T. T., Taya, Y., Thorgeirsson, S. S., et al. (2002) Cyclin G recruits PP2A to dephosphorylate Mdm2. *Mol. Cell* **9**, 761–771.

139. Kimura, S. H., Ikawa, M., Ito, A., Okabe, M., and Nojima, H. (2001) Cyclin G1 is involved in G2/M arrest in response to DNA damage and in growth control after damage recovery. *Oncogene* **20**, 3290–3300.

140. Ito, A., Kataoka, T. R., Watanabe, M., Nishiyama, K., Mazaki, Y., Sabe, H., et al. (2000) A truncated isoform of the PP2A B56 subunit promotes cell motility through paxillin phosphorylation. *EMBO J.* 19, 562–571.

141. Ito, A., Koma, Y., Watabe, K., Nagano, T., Endo, Y., Nojima, H., et al. (2003) A truncated isoform of the protein phosphatase 2A B56gamma regulatory subunit may promote genetic instability and cause tumor progression. *Am. J. Pathol.* **162**, 81–91.

142. Zhao, L., Samuels, T., Winckler, S., Korgaonkar, C., Tompkins, V., Horne, M.C., et al. (2003) Cyclin G1 has growth inhibitory activity linked to the ARF-Mdm2-p53 and pRb tumor suppressor pathways. *Mol. Cancer Res.* **1**, 195–206.

143. Lowndes, N. F. and Murguia, J. R. (2000) Sensing and responding to DNA damage. *Curr. Opin. Genet. Dev.* **10**, 17–25.

144. Naiki, T., Shimomura, T., Kondo, T., Matsumoto, K., and Sugimoto, K. (2000) Rfc5, in cooperation with rad24, controls DNA damage checkpoints throughout the cell cycle in *Saccharomyces cerevisiae. Mol. Cell Biol.* **20,** 5888–5896.
145. Shimada, M., Okuzaki, D., Tanaka, S., Tougan, T., Yoneki, T., Tamai, K. K., et al. (1999) Replication factor C of *S. pombe,* a small subunit of replication factor complex, plays a role in both replication and damage checkpoints. *Mol. Biol. Cell* **10,** 3991–4003.
146. O'Connell, M. J., Walworth, N, C., and Carr, A. M. (2000) The G2-phase DNA-damage checkpoint. *Trends Cell Biol.* **10,** 296–303.
147. Majka, J. and Burgers, P. M. (2003) Yeast Rad17/Mec3/Ddc1: a sliding clamp for the DNA damage checkpoint. *Proc. Natl. Acad. Sci. USA* **100,** 2249–2254.
148. Walworth, N., Davey, S., and Beach, D. (1993) Fission yeast chk1 protein kinase links the rad checkpoint pathway to cdc2. *Nature* **363,** 368–371.
149. Carr, A. M. (2002) DNA structure dependent checkpoints as regulators of DNA repair. *DNA Repair (Amst)* **1,** 983–994.
150. Tzivion, G., Shen, Y. H., and Zhu, J. (2001) 14-3-3 proteins; bringing new definitions to scaffolding. *Oncogene* **20,** 6331–6338.
151. Melo, J. and Toczyski, D. (2002) A unified view of the DNA-damage checkpoint. *Curr. Opin. Cell Biol.* **14,** 237–245.
152. Sanchez, Y., Wong, C., Thoma, R. S., Richman, R., Wu, Z., Piwnica-Worms, H., et al. (1997) Conservation of the Chk1 checkpoint pathway in mammals: linkage of DNA damage to Cdk regulation through Cdc25. *Science* **277,** 1497–1501
153. Peng, C. Y., Graves, P. R., Thoma, R. S., Wu, Z., Shaw, A., and Piwnica-Worms, H. (1997) Mitotic and G$_2$ checkpoint control: regulation of 14-3-3 protein binding by phosphorylation of Cdc25C on serine-216. *Science* **277,** 1501–1505.
154. Walworth, N. C. (2000) Cell-cycle checkpoint kinases: checking in on the cell cycle. *Curr. Opin. Cell Biol.* **12,** 697–704.
155. Bartek, J. and Lukas, J. (2003) Chk1 and Chk2 kinases in checkpoint control and cancer. *Cancer Cell* **3,** 421–429.
156. Chen, M. J., Lin, Y. T., Lieberman, H. B., Chen, G., and Lee, E. Y. (2001) ATM-dependent phosphorylation of human Rad9 is required for ionizing radiation–induced checkpoint activation *J. Biol. Chem.* **276,** 16580–16586.
157. Bahassi, el M., Conn, C. W., Myer, D. L., Hennigan, R. F., McGowan, C. H., Sanchez, Y., et al. (2002) Mammalian Polo-like kinase 3 (Plk3) is a multifunctional protein involved in stress response pathways. *Oncogene* **21,** 6633–6640.
158. Yazdi, P. T., Wang, Y., Zhao, S., Patel, N., Lee, E. Y., and Qin, J. (2002) SMC1 is a downstream effector in the ATM/NBS1 branch of the human S-phase checkpoint. *Genes Dev.* **16,** 571–582.
159. Kim, S. T., Xu, B., and Kastan, M. B. (2002) Involvement of the cohesin protein, Smc1, in Atm-dependent and independent responses to DNA damage. *Genes Dev.* **16,** 560–570.

160. Fernandez-Capetillo, O., Chen, H. T., Celeste, A., Ward, I., Romanienko, P. J., Morales, J. C., et al. (2002) DNA damage–induced G2-M checkpoint activation by histone H2AX and 53BP1. *Nat. Cell Biol.* **4**, 993–997.

161. Ward, I. M., Minn, K., Jorda, K. G., and Chen, J. (2003) Accumulation of checkpoint protein 53BP1 at DNA breaks involves its binding to phosphorylated histone H2AX. *J. Biol. Chem.* **278**, 19579–19582.

162. Goldberg, M., Stucki, M., Falck, J., D'Amours, D., Rahman, D., Pappin, D., et al. (2003) MDC1 is required for the intra-S-phase DNA damage checkpoint. *Nature* **421**, 952–956.

163. Cortez, D., Guntuku, S., Qin, J., and Elledge, S. J. (2001) ATR and ATRIP: partners in checkpoint signaling. *Science* **294**, 1713–1716.

164. Edwards, R. J., Bentley, N. J., and Carr, A. M. (1999) A Rad3–Rad26 complex responds to DNA damage independently of other checkpoint proteins. *Nat. Cell Biol.* **1**, 393–398.

165. Paciotti, V., Clerici, M., Lucchini, G., and Longhese, M. P. (2000) The checkpoint protein Ddc2, functionally related to *S. pombe* Rad26, interacts with Mec1 and is regulated by Mec1-dependent phosphorylation in budding yeast. *Genes Dev.* **14**, 2046–2059.

166. Rouse, J. and Jackson, S. P. (2000) LCD1: an essential gene involved in checkpoint control and regulation of the MEC1 signalling pathway in *Saccharomyces cerevisiae*. *EMBO J.* **19**, 5801–5812.

167. Wakayama, T., Kondo, T., Ando, S., Matsumoto, K., and Sugimoto, K. (2001) Pie1, a protein interacting with Mec1, controls cell growth and checkpoint responses in *Saccharomyces cerevisiae*. *Mol. Cell. Biol.* **21**, 755–764.

168. Ward, I. M. and Chen, J. (2001) Histone H2AX is phosphorylated in an ATR-dependent manner in response to replicational stress. *J. Biol. Chem.* **276**, 47759–47762.

169. Lin, W. C., Lin, F. T., and Nevins, J. R. (2001) Selective induction of E2F1 in response to DNA damage, mediated by ATM-dependent phosphorylation. *Genes Dev.* **15**, 1833–1844.

170. McGowan, C. H. (2002) Checking in on Cds1 (Chk2): A checkpoint kinase and tumor suppressor. *Bioessays* **24**, 502–511.

171. Gatei, M., Sloper, K., Sorensen, C., Syljuasen, R., Falck, J., Hobson, K., et al. (2003) *Ataxia-telangiectasia*-mutated (ATM) and NBS1-dependent phosphorylation of Chk1 on Ser-317 in response to ionizing radiation. *J. Biol. Chem.* **278**, 14806–14811.

172. Groth, A., Lukas, J., Nigg, E. A., Sillje, H. H., Wernstedt, C., Bartek, J., et al. (2003) Human Tousled like kinases are targeted by an ATM- and Chk1-dependent DNA damage checkpoint. *EMBO J.* **22**, 1676–1687.

173. Lukas, C., Falck, J., Bartkova, J., Bartek, J., and Lukas, J. (2003) Distinct spatiotemporal dynamics of mammalian checkpoint regulators induced by DNA damage. *Nat. Cell Biol.* **5**, 255–260.

174. Zhao, H. and Piwnica-Worms, H. (2001) ATR-mediated checkpoint pathways regulate phosphorylation and activation of human Chk1. *Mol. Cell. Biol.* **21**, 4129–4139.

175. Liu, Q., Guntuku, S., Cui, X. S., Matsuoka, S., Cortez, D., Tamai, K., et al. (2000) Chk1 is an essential kinase that is regulated by Atr and required for the G(2)/M DNA damage checkpoint. *Genes Dev.* **14,** 1448–1459.

176. Bulavin, D. V., Amundson, S. A., and Fornace, A. J. (2002) P38 and Chk1 kinases: different conductors for the G(2)/M checkpoint symphony. *Curr. Opin. Genet. Dev.* **12,** 92–97.

177. Jiang, K., Pereira, E., Maxfield, M., Russell, B., Goudelock, D. M., and Sanchez, Y. (2003) Regulation of Chk1 includes chromatin association and 14-3-3 binding following phosphorylation on Ser345. *J. Biol. Chem.* **278,** 25207–25217.

178. Goudelock, D. M., Jiang, K., Pereira, E., Russell, B., and Sanchez, Y. (2003) Regulatory interactions between the checkpoint kinase Chk1 and the proteins of the DNA-PK complex. *J. Biol. Chem.* **278,** 29940–29947.

179. Li, S., Ting, N. S., Zheng, L., Chen, P. L., Ziv, Y., Shiloh, Y., et al. (2000) Functional link of BRCA1 and ataxia telangiectasia gene product in DNA damage response. *Nature* **406,** 210–215.

180. Takai, H., Tominaga, K., Motoyama, N., Minamishima, Y. A., Nagahama, H., Tsukiyama, T., et al. (2000) Aberrant cell cycle checkpoint function and early embryonic death in Chk1$^{-/-}$ mice. *Genes Dev.* **14,** 1439–1447.

181. Zachos, G., Rainey, M. D., and Gillespie, D. A. (2003) Chk1-deficient tumour cells are viable but exhibit multiple checkpoint and survival defects. *EMBO J.* **22,** 713–723.

182. Matsuoka, S., Rotman, G., Ogawa, A., Shiloh, Y., Tamai, K., and Elledge, S. J. (2000) *Ataxia telangiectasia*–mutated phosphorylates Chk2 in vivo and in vitro. *Proc. Natl. Acad. Sci. USA* **97,** 10389–10394.

183. Hirao, A., Cheung, A., Duncan, G., Girard, P. M., Elia, A. J., Wakeham, A., et al. (2002) Chk2 is a tumor suppressor that regulates apoptosis in both an ataxia telangiectasia mutated (ATM)-dependent and an ATM-independent manner. *Mol. Cell Biol.* **22,** 6521–6532.

184. Takai, H., Naka, K., Okada ,Y., Watanabe, M., Harada, N., Saito, S., et al. (2002) Chk2-deficient mice exhibit radioresistance and defective p53-mediated transcription. *EMBO J.* **21,** 5195–5205.

185. Boddy, M. N., Lopez-Girona, A., Shanahan, P., Interthal, H., Heyer, W. D., and Russell, P. (2000) Damage tolerance protein Mus81 associates with the FHA1 domain of checkpoint kinase Cds1. *Mol. Cell Biol.* **20,** 8758–8766.

186. Boddy, M. N., Gaillard, P. H., McDonald, W. H., Shanahan, P., Yates, J. R., 3rd, and Russell, P. (2001) Mus81-Eme1 are essential components of a Holliday junction resolvase. *Cell* **107,** 537–548.

187. Ciccia, A., Constantinou, A., and West, S. C. (2003) Identification and characterization of the human mus81-eme1 endonuclease. *J. Biol. Chem.* **278,** 25172–25178.

188. Xie, S., Wu, H., Wang, Q., Kunicki, J., Thomas, R. O., Hollingsworth, R. E., et al. (2002) Genotoxic stress-induced activation of Plk3 is partly mediated by Chk2. *Cell Cycle* **1,** 424–429.

189. Yang, H., Jeffrey, P. D., Miller, J., Kinnucan, E., Sun, Y., Thoma, N. H., et al. (2002) BRCA2 function in DNA binding and recombination from a BRCA2-DSS1-ssDNA structure. *Science* **297,**1837–1848.

190. Stevens, C., Smith, L., and LaThangue, N. B. (2003) Chk2 activates E2F-1 in response to DNA damage. *Nat. Cell Biol.* **5**, 401–409.

191. Louria-Hayon, I., Grossman, T., Sionov, R. V., Alsheich, O., Pandolfi, P. P., and Haupt, Y. (2003) PML protects p53 from Mdm2-mediated inhibition and degradation. *J. Biol. Chem.* **278**, 33134–33141.

192. Roe, J. L., Nemhauser, J. L., and Zambryski, P. C. (1997) TOUSLED participates in apical tissue formation during gynoecium development in *Arabidopsis. Plant Cell* **9**, 335–353.

193. Silljé, H. H. W. and Nigg, E. A. (2001) Identification of human Asf1 chromatin assembly factors as substrates of Tousled-like kinases. *Curr. Biol.* **11**, 1068–1073.

194. Pardee, A. B. (1974) A restriction point for control of normal animal cell proliferation. *Proc. Natl. Acad. Sci. USA* **71**, 1286–1290.

195. Pardee, A. B. (1989) G1 events and regulation of cell proliferation. *Science* **246**, 603–608.

196. Blagosklonny, M. V. and Pardee, A. B. (2002) The restriction point of the cell cycle. *Cell Cycle* **1**, 103–110.

197. Bartek, J. and Lukas, J. (2001) Mammalian G1- and S-phase checkpoints in response to DNA damage. *Curr. Opin. Cell Biol.* **13**, 738–747.

198. Zhao, H. and Piwnica-Worms, H. (2001) ATR-mediated checkpoint pathways regulate phosphorylation and activation of human Chk1. *Mol. Cell. Biol.* **21**, 4129–4139.

199. Kastan, M. B. and Lim, D. S. (2000) The many substrates and functions of ATM. *Nat. Rev. Mol. Cell Biol.* **1**, 179–186.

200. Takisawa, H., Mimura, S., and Kubota, Y. (2000) Eukaryotic DNA replication: from pre-replication complex to initiation complex. *Curr. Opin. Cell Biol.* **12**, 690–696.

201. Lei, M. and Tye, B. K. (2001) Initiating DNA synthesis: from recruiting to activating the MCM complex. *J. Cell Sci.* **114**, 1447–1454.

202. Falck, J., Lukas, C., Protopopova, M., Lukas, J., Selivanova, G., and Bartek, J. (2001) Functional impact of concomitant versus alternative defects in the Chk2-p53 tumour suppressor pathway. *Oncogene* **20**, 5503–5510.

203. Ducruet, A. P. and Lazo, J. S. (2003) Regulation of Cdc25A half-life in interphase by cyclin-dependent kinase 2 activity. *J. Biol. Chem.* **278**, 31838–31842.

204. Agami, R. and Bernars, R. (2000) Distinct initiation and maintenance mechanisms cooperate to induce G1 cell cycle arrest in response to DNA damage. *Cell* **102**, 55–66.

205. Labib, K., Kearsey, S. E., and Diffley, J. F. (2001) MCM2-7 proteins are essential components of prereplicative complexes that accumulate cooperatively in the nucleus during G1-phase and are required to establish, but not maintain, the S-phase checkpoint. *Mol. Biol. Cell* **12**, 3658–3667.

206. Kubota, Y., Mimura, S., Nishimoto, S., Takisawa, A., and Nojima, H. (1995) Identification of the yeast MCM3 related protein as a component of *Xenopus* DNA replication licensing factor. *Cell* **81**, 601–609.

207. Hingorani, M. M. and O'Donnell, M. (2000) A tale of toroids in DNA metabolism. *Nat. Rev. Mol. Cell Biol.* **1,** 22–30.

208. Yabuta, N., Kajimura, N., Mayanagi, K., Sato, M., Gotow, T., Uchiyama, Y., et al. (2003) Mammalian Mcm2/4/6/7 complex forms a toroidal structure. *Genes Cells* **8,** 413–421.

209. Masai, H. and Arai, K. (2002) Cdc7 kinase complex: a key regulator in the initiation of DNA replication. *J. Cell Physiol.* **190,** 287–296.

210. Shreeram, S., Sparks, A., Lane, D. P., and Blow, J. J. (2002) Cell type–specific responses of human cells to inhibition of replication licensing. *Oncogene* **21,** 6624–6632.

211. Tercero, J. A. and Diffley, J. F. (2001) Regulation of DNA replication fork progression through damaged DNA by the Mec1/Rad53 checkpoint. *Nature* **412,** 553–557.

212. Tercero, J. A. and Diffley, J. F. (2003) A central role for DNA replication forks in checkpoint activation and response. *Mol. Cell* **11,** 1323–1336.

213. Wang, H. and Elledge, S. J. (1999) DRC1, DNA replication and checkpoint protein 1, functions with DPB11 to control DNA replication and the S-phase checkpoint in *Saccharomyces cerevisiae. Proc. Natl. Acad. Sci. USA* **96,** 3824–3829.

214. Wang, H. and Elledge, S. J. (2002) Genetic and physical interactions between DPB11 and DDC1 in the yeast DNA damage response pathway. *Genetics* **160,** 1295–1304.

215. Mäkiniemi, M., Hillukkala, T., Tuusa, J., Reini, K., Vaara, M., Huang, D., et al. (2001) BRCT domain-containing protein TopBP1 functions in DNA replication and damage response. *J. Biol. Chem.* **276,** 30399–30406.

216. You, Z., Kong, L., and Newport, J. (2002) The role of single-stranded DNA and Pol α in establishing the ATR, Hus1 DNA replication checkpoint. *J. Biol. Chem.* **277,** 27088–27093.

217. Kumagai, A. and Dunphy, W. G. (2000) Claspin, a novel protein required for the activation of Chk1 during a DNA replication checkpoint response in *Xenopus* egg extracts. *Mol. Cell* **6,** 839–849.

218. Lee, J., Kumagai, A., and Dunphy, W. G. (2003) Claspin, a Chk1-regulatory protein, monitors DNA replication on chromatin independently of RPA, ATR, and Rad17. *Mol. Cell* **11,** 329–340.

219. Kumagai, A. and Dunphy, W. G. (2003) Repeated phosphopeptide motifs in Claspin mediate the regulated binding of Chk1. *Nat. Cell Biol.* **5,** 161–165.

220. Chini, C. C. and Chen, J. (2003) Human Claspin is required for replication checkpoint control. *J. Biol. Chem.* **278,** 30057–30062.

221. Gilbert, C. S., Green, C. M., and Lowndes, N. F. (2001) Budding yeast Rad9 is an ATP-dependent Rad53 activating machine. *Mol. Cell* **8,** 129–136.

222. Alcasabas, A. A., Osborn, A. J., Hu, F., Werler, P. J., Bousset, K., Fukuya, K., et al. (2001) Mrc1 transduces signals of DNA replication stress to activate Rad53. *Nat. Cell Biol.* **3,** 958–965.

223. Tanaka, K. and Russell, P. (2001) Mrc1 channels the DNA replication arrest signal to checkpoint kinase Cds1. *Nat. Cell Biol.* **3,** 966–972.

224. Shimada, K., Pasero, P., and Gasser, S. M. (2002) ORC and the intra-S-phase checkpoint: a threshold regulates Rad53p activation in S phase. *Genes Dev.* **16,** 3236–3252.

225. Choy, J. S. and Kron, S. J. (2002) NuA4 subunit Yng2 function in intra-S-phase DNA damage response. *Mol. Cell Biol.* **22,** 8215–8225.

226. Marchetti, M. A., Kumar, S., Hartsuiker, E., Maftahi, M., Carr, A. M., Freyer, G. A., et al. (2002) A single unbranched S-phase DNA damage and replication fork blockage checkpoint pathway. *Proc. Natl. Acad. Sci. USA* **99,** 7472–7477.

227. Falck, J., Petrini, J. H., Williams, B. R., Lukas, J., and Bartek, J. (2002) The DNA damage–dependent intra-S phase checkpoint is regulated by parallel pathways. *Nat. Genet.* **30,** 290–294.

228. Cortez, D., Wang, Y., Qin, J., and Elledge, S. J. (1999) Requirement of ATM-dependent phosphorylation of BRCA1 in the DNA damage response to double-strand breaks. *Science* **286,** 1162–1166.

229. Li, S., Ting, N. S., Zheng, L., Chen, P. L., Ziv, Y., Shiloh, Y., et al. (2000) Functional link of BRCA1 and ataxia telangiectasia gene product in DNA damage response. *Nature* **406,** 210–215.

230. Moynahan, M. E. (2002) The cancer connection: BRCA1 and BRCA2 tumor suppression in mice and humans. *Oncogene* **21,** 8994–9007.

231. Brodie, S. G. and Deng, C. X. (2001) BRCA1-associated tumorigenesis: what have we learned from knockout mice? *Trends Genet.* **17,** S18–S22.

232. D'Andrea, A. D. and Grompe, M. (2003) The Fanconi anaemia/BRCA pathway. *Nat. Rev. Cancer* **3,** 23–34.

233. Yang, S., Kuo, C., Bisi, J. E., and Kim, M. K. (2002) PML-dependent apoptosis after DNA damage is regulated by the checkpoint kinase hCds1/Chk2. *Nat. Cell Biol.* **4,** 865–870.

234. Wu, X., Ranganathan, V., Weisman, D. S., Heine, W. F., Ciccone, D. N., O'Neill, T. B., et al. (2000) ATM phosphorylation of Nijmegen breakage syndrome protein is required in a DNA damage response. *Nature* **405,** 477–482

235. Zhao, S., Weng, Y. C., Yuan, S. S., Lin, Y. T., Hsu, H. C., Lin, S. C., et al. (2000) Functional link between ataxia-telangiectasia and Nijmegen breakage syndrome gene products. *Nature* **405,** 473–477.

236. Gatei, M., Young, D., Cerosaletti, K. M., Desai-Mehta, A., Spring, K., Kozlov, S., et al. (2000) ATM-dependent phosphorylation of nibrin in response to radiation exposure. *Nat. Genet.* **25,** 115–119.

237. D'Amours, D. and Jackson, S. P. (2002) The Mre11 complex: at the crossroads of DNA repair and checkpoint signaling. *Nat. Rev. Mol. Cell Biol.* **3,** 317–327.

238. Lim, D. S., Kim, S. T., Xu, B., Maser, R. S., Lin, J., Petrini, J. H., et al. (2000) ATM phosphorylates p95/nbs1 in an S-phase checkpoint pathway. *Nature* **404,** 613–617.

239. Petrini, J. H. (2000) The Mre11 complex and ATM: collaborating to navigate S phase. *Curr. Opin. Cell Biol.* **12,** 293–296.

240. Tauchi, H., Matsuura, S., Kobayashi, J., Sakamoto, S., and Komatsu, K. (2002) Nijmegen breakage syndrome gene, NBS1, and molecular links to factors for genome stability. *Oncogene* **21,** 8967–8980.

241. Wang, H., Wang, X., Zhou, X. Y., Chen, D. J., Li, G. C., Iliakis, G., et al. (2002) Ku affects the ataxia and Rad 3–related/CHK1-dependent S phase checkpoint response after camptothecin treatment. *Cancer Res.* **62**, 2483–2487.

242. Feijoo, C., Hall-Jackson, C., Wu, R., Jenkins, D., Leitch, J., Gilbert, D. M., et al. (2001) Activation of mammalian Chk1 during DNA replication arrest: a role for Chk1 in the intra-S phase checkpoint monitoring replication origin firing. *J. Cell Biol.* **154**, 913–923.

243. Cliby, W. A., Lewis, K. A., Lilly, K. K., and Kaufmann, S. H. (2002) S phase and G_2 arrests induced by topoisomerase I poisons are dependent on ATR kinase function. *J. Biol. Chem.* **277**, 1599–1606.

244. Wang, B., Matsuoka, S., Carpenter, P. B., and Elledge, S. J. (2002) 53BP1, a mediator of the DNA damage checkpoint. *Science* **298**, 1435–1438.

245. Redon, C., Pilch, D. R., Rogakou, E. P., Orr, A. H., Lowndes, N. F., and Bonner, W. M. (2003) Yeast histone 2A serine 129 is essential for the efficient repair of checkpoint-blind DNA damage. *EMBO Rep.* **4**, 1–7.

246. Costanzo, V., Shechter, D., Lupardus, P. J., Cimprich, K. A., Gottesman, M., and Gautier, J. (2003) An ATR- and Cdc7-dependent DNA damage checkpoint that inhibits initiation of DNA replication. *Mol. Cell.* **11**, 203–213.

247. Stewart, G. S., Wang, B., Bignell, C. R., Taylor, A. M., and Elledge, S. J. (2003) MDC1 is a mediator of the mammalian DNA damage checkpoint. *Nature* **421**, 961–966.

248. Canman, C. E. (2003) Checkpoint mediators: relaying signals from DNA strand breaks. *Curr. Biol.* **13**, R488–R490.

249. Goldberg, M., Stucki, M., Falck, J., D'Amours, D., Rahman, D., Pappin, D., et al. (2003) MDC1 is required for the intra-S-phase DNA damage checkpoint. *Nature* **421**, 952–956.

250. Hubscher, U., Maga, G. and Spadari, S. (2002) Eukaryotic DNA polymerases. *Annu. Rev. Biochem.* **71**, 133–163.

251. Lindsey-Boltz, L. A., Bermudez, V. P., Hurwitz, J., and Sancar, A. (2001) Purification and characterization of human DNA damage checkpoint Rad complexes. *Proc. Natl. Acad. Sci. USA* **98**, 11236–11241.

252. Melo, J. A., Cohen, J., and Toczyski, D. P. (2001) Two checkpoint complexes are independently recruited to sites of DNA damage in vivo. *Genes Dev.* **15**, 2809–2821.

253. Kondo, T., Wakayama, T., Naiki, T., Matsumoto, K., and Sugimoto, K. (2001) Recruitment of Mec1 and Ddc1 checkpoint proteins to double-strand breaks through distinct mechanisms. *Science* **294**, 867–870.

254. Zou, L., Cortez, D., and Elledge, S. J. (2002) Regulation of ATR substrate selection by Rad17-dependent loading of Rad9 complexes onto chromatin. *Genes Dev.* **16**, 198–208.

255. Weiss, R. S., Matsuoka, S., Elledge, S. J., and Leder, P. (2002) Hus1 acts upstream of chk1 in a mammalian DNA damage response pathway. *Curr. Biol.* **12**, 73–77.

256. Bao, S., Tibbetts, R. S., Brumbaugh, K. M., Fang, Y., Richardson, D. A., Ali, A., et al. (2001) ATR/ATM-mediated phosphorylation of human Rad17 is required for genotoxic stress responses. *Nature* **411**, 969–974.

257. Weiss, R. S., Leder, P., and Vaziri, C. (2003) Critical role for mouse Hus1 in an S-phase DNA damage cell cycle checkpoint. *Mol. Cell Biol.* **23**, 791–803.

258. Varley, J. (2003) TP53, hChk2, and the Li-Fraumeni syndrome. *Methods Mol. Biol.* **222**, 117–29.

259. Sharpless, E. and Chin, L. (2003) The INK4a/ARF locus and melanoma. *Oncogene* **22**, 3092–3098.

260. Lindstrom, M. S. and Wiman, K. G. (2002) Role of genetic and epigenetic changes in Burkitt lymphoma. *Semin. Cancer Biol.* **12**, 381–387.

261. Cangi, M. G., Cukor, B., Soung, P., Signoretti, S., Moreira, G.., Ranashinge, M., Jr., et al. (2000) Role of the Cdc25A phosphatase in human breast cancer. *J. Clin. Invest.* **106**, 753–761.

262. Shiloh, Y. (2001) ATM and ATR: networking cellular responses to DNA damage. *Curr. Opin. Genet. Dev.* **11**, 71–77.

263. Bell, D. W., Varley, J. M., Szydlo, T. E., Kang, D. H., Wahrer, D. C., Shannon, K. E., et al. (1999) Heterozygous germ line hCHK2 mutations in Li-Fraumeni syndrome. *Science* **286**, 2528–2531.

264. Stewart, G. S., Maser, R. S., Stankovic, T., Bressan, D. A., Kaplan, M. I., Jaspers, N. G., et al. (1999) The DNA double-strand break repair gene hMRE11 is mutated in individuals with an ataxia-telangiectasia-like disorder. *Cell* **99**, 577–587.

265. Bagby, G. C., Jr. (2003) Genetic basis of Fanconi anemia. *Curr. Opin. Hematol.* **10**, 68–76.

266. Tischkowitz, M. D. and Hodgson, S. V. (2003) Fanconi anaemia. *J. Med. Genet.* **40**, 1–10.

267. Taniguchi, T., Garcia-Higuera, I., Andreassen, P. R., Gregory, R. C., Grompe, M., and D'Andrea, A. D. (2002) S-phase-specific interaction of the Fanconi anemia protein, FANCD2, with BRCA1 and RAD51. *Blood* **100**, 2414–2420.

268. Taniguchi, T., Garcia-Higuera, I., Xu, B., Andreassen, P. R., Gregory, R. C., Kim, S. T., et al. (2002) Convergence of the Fanconi anemia and ataxia telangiectasia signaling pathways. *Cell* **109**, 459–472.

269. Venkitaraman, A. R. (2002) Cancer susceptibility and the functions of BRCA1 and BRCA2. *Cell* **108**, 171–182.

270. Scully, R. and Livingston, D. M. (2000) In search of the tumour-suppressor functions of BRCA1 and BRCA2. *Nature* **408**, 429–432.

271. Pagano, G. and Youssoufian, H. (2003) Fanconi anaemia proteins: major roles in cell protection against oxidative damage. *Bioessays* **25**, 589–595.

272. Xu, X., Aprelikova, O., Moens, P., Deng, C. X., and Furth, P. A. (2003) Impaired meiotic DNA-damage repair and lack of crossing-over during spermatogenesis in BRCA1 full-length isoform deficient mice. *Development* **130**, 2001–2012.

273. Ababou, M., Dutertre, S., Lecluse, Y., Onclercq, R., Chatton, B., and Amor-Gueret, M. (2000) ATM-dependent phosphorylation and accumulation of endogenous BLM protein in response to ionizing radiation. *Oncogene* **19**, 5955–5963.

274. Ababou, M., Dumaire, V., Lecluse, Y., and Amor-Gueret, M. (2002) Bloom's

syndrome protein response to ultraviolet-C radiation and hydroxyurea-mediated DNA synthesis inhibition. *Oncogene* **21**, 2079–2088.

275. Lange, B. M. (2002) Integration of the centrosome in cell cycle control, stress response and signal transduction pathways. *Curr. Opin. Cell Biol.* **14**, 35–43.

276. Nigg, E. A. (2002) Centrosome aberrations: cause or consequence of cancer progression? *Nat. Rev. Cancer* **2**, 815–825.

277. Tarapore, P. and Fukasawa, K. (2002) Loss of p53 and centrosome hyperamplification. *Oncogene* **21**, 6234–6240.

characterized by lengthening of a cell cycle phase, but also to a "wee" phenotype characterized by the shortening of the cell cycle and division at a smaller size *(5)*. Additional studies with *S. pombe* uncovered *cdc25* and *wee1*, and indicated that *cdc25* encoded an activator of the *cdc2* gene product, while *wee1* encoded an inhibitor *(6–8)*. The isolation of *wee1* mutants was significant because *wee1* is a gene whose inactivation caused acceleration of the cell cycle, and encoded an inhibitor of a rate-limiting process. Cdc mutants, on the other hand, could map to any gene that was required for cell cycle progression, not necessarily part of the regulatory network.

Studies in yeast involving ingenious and laborious genetic screens laid important groundwork for the analysis of the G2 phase. Equally amazing was the convergence of experimental approaches that allowed the realization that the same protein could control entry into mitosis in yeast, mammals, frogs, starfish, and many other organisms. Studies in the large oocytes of frogs and starfish identified a factor that could induce entry into mitosis when microinjected, called maturation promoting factor (MPF) *(9–11)*. The components of MPF were not to be identified for many years. One problem was that the high concentration of MPF required to induce mitosis using microinjection precluded its purification. This problem was overcome with the development of cell-free extracts that recapitulated many of the mitotic processes when MPF was added *(12–14)*. Highly purified MPF was found to contain two proteins of molecular weight 34 and 45 kDa *(15)*. Immunoblotting and immunoprecipitation using antibodies raised against the *S. pombe cdc2* gene product were used to show that the 34 kDa subunit was identical to Cdc2 *(16,17)*. *S. pombe* Cdc2 was known to bind to the product of the *suc1* gene, which was exploited to show that MPF could be depleted using Suc1 purified from bacteria and immobilized on agarose beads *(18,19)*. This result added further evidence that MPF contained Cdc2.

A separate line of investigation resolved the identity of the 45 kDa component of MPF. Sea urchin oocytes were found to contain proteins that oscillated during the cell cycle with highest levels in mitosis; these are called *cyclins* *(20)*. *cyclin* mRNA could induce entry in mitosis when injected into frog oocytes, and was the only mRNA needed to drive a frog oocyte extract into mitosis *(21–23)*. Subsequent western blotting and immunoprecipitation studies with antibodies raised against frog cyclin proved that the 45kDa subunit of MPF was a cyclin *(24)*. This was consistent with studies documenting the interaction between p34Cdc2 and cyclins in the clam *Spisula solidissima (25)*.

Additional proof for a universal controller of mitosis came from studies of histone phosphorylation. The growth-associated H1 histone kinase was observed to vary during the cell cycle in many types of cells, including sea urchin, starfish and frog oocytes, and mammalian fibroblasts, and the highest levels of activity were detected in mitosis *(26–30)*. Interestingly, a partially purified H1 kinase could accelerate mitosis in *Physarium*, leading the authors to suggest that their H1 kinase was a conserved regulator of mitotic entry *(31)*. The identification of the H1 kinase as the product of the *cdc2* gene was made many years later, using a combination of chromatographic purification and an antibody against the cloned *cdc2* gene product *(18)*. The realization that Cdc2 is a conserved inducer of mitosis illustrates an important idea in cell cycle research. By combining a diversity of methods and using information from diverse organisms, considerable progress was made.

2. Our Current Understanding of Cdc2 Regulation

Many of the regulatory steps that control Cdc2 activity have been elucidated and have been conserved during evolution, although some details are different (reviewed in *32,33*). Cdc2 is active only at the G2/M border and is turned off as cells enter the anaphase stage of mitosis. The first step in generating active Cdc2 is its association with a cyclin (**Fig. 1**). In animal cells, Cdc2 associates with an A-type or a B-type cyclin, in fission yeast with Cdc13, and in budding yeast with the CLB proteins. The cyclins that bind to Cdc2 accumulate as cells progress through G2 and are degraded when cells progress from metaphase to anaphase, thus extinguishing Cdc2 kinase activity.

During G2, Cdc2/cyclin B is actively excluded from the nucleus, where it must go to phosphorylate the substrates that will bring about the various steps of mitosis *(34–36)*. During G2, the Cdc2–cyclin B1 complex is kept in the cytoplasm by nuclear export, mediated by binding of the cyclin subunit to the exportin protein CRM1 *(34,36,37)* (**Fig. 1**). Export by Crm1 counterbalances the constitutive import of the complex mediated by binding of the cyclin subunit to importin β *(38,39)*. As cells approach the G2/M boundary, cyclin B1 becomes phosphorylated in its Crm1 binding site, which blocks binding and stops export, allowing the accumulation of the Cdc2–cyclin B complex in the nucleus, where it can induce entry into mitosis *(37)* (**Fig. 1**). The Crm1 binding site of cyclin B can be phosphorylated by Cdc2 and also by Plk1, an enzyme found in many organisms including *Drosophila*, frogs, and yeast, and known to be required for multiple events during mitosis *(40–42)*.

Cdc2 must be phosphorylated at threonine 161 to be active, and in animal cells this process is catalyzed by cyclin-dependent kinase (CDK)-activating kinase (CAK) *(43,44)* (**Fig. 1**) . As animal cells approach the G2/M boundary, the accumulating Cdc2–cyclin B complex is kept inactive by two inhibitory phosphorylations on the Cdc2 subunit at tyrosine 15, catalyzed by Wee1, and at threonine 14, catalyzed by Myt1 *(45–47)* (**Fig. 1**). In fission yeast, only the conserved tyrosine residue is phosphorylated to turn off the kinase *(48)*. In budding yeast, although the conserved tyrosine of Cdc28 is phosphorylated, this is not an important factor in the regulation of the kinase *(49,50)*.

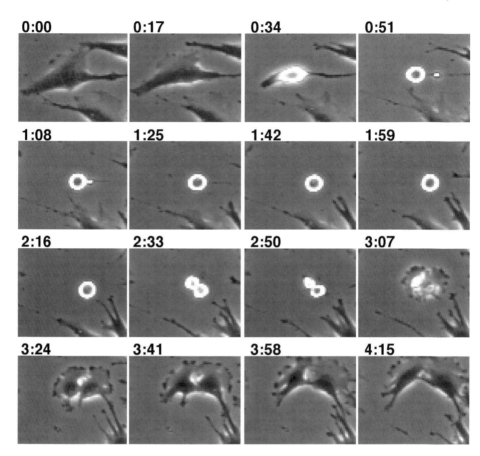

Fig. 3. Time-lapse images of the mitotic process. Phase contrast images of a human fibroblast entering and progressing through mitosis are shown. An image was taken every 17 min. By viewing approx 100 cells at a time, the mitotic activity of a culture can be assessed over time.

logical functions, including Bax, Puma, Pig3, and Noxa, which are important in inducing apoptosis, and p21/waf1, Gadd45, and 14-3-3σ, which are inducers of growth arrest *(116)*. p21/waf1 is a major target of p53 that is essential for G1 arrest. Unlike yeast, in which Cdc2 can control both the G1/S and G2/M transitions, mammalian cells have a family of kinases with homology to Cdc2. These kinases require a cyclin subunit for activity, are called cyclin-dependent kinases (CDKs), and control the major mammalian cell cycle transitions. p21/ waf1 is an efficient inhibitor of CDK2, 4, and 6, which explains its ability to block cells at the G1/S boundary *(133)*. p21/waf1 can bind only poorly to Cdc2, yet can arrest cells in G2 when overexpressed *(133–136)*. In addition, HCT116 cells lacking p21/waf1 arrest only transiently in G2 in response to adriamycin, adding further support for the involvement of this protein in stabilizing G2 arrest *(132)*. One mechanism that has been proposed for G2 arrest by p21/waf1 involves its ability to block the activating phosphorylation of Cdc2 at threonine 161, but the mechanism by which p21/waf1 reduces this phosphorylation is not known *(137)*. Our work has uncovered an additional mechanism by which p21/waf1 contributes to the stability of G2 arrest.

Gadd45 has also been implicated in G2 arrest induced by p53. Gadd45 can bind to Cdc2 and dissociate the cyclin B subunit, thus inactivating the complex *(138,139)*. The G2 delay that occurs in response to ultraviolet radiation is reduced in lymphocytes when Gadd45 is deleted *(140)*. The 14-3-3σ target of p53 can cause G2 arrest when overexpressed *(141)*. It appears to do so by binding to the Cdc2–cyclin B complex and anchoring it in the cytoplasm, where it is unable to induce mitosis *(142)*. Deletion of 14-3-3σ from HCT116 cells caused the cells to escape from the G2 arrest induced by adriamycin and enter mitosis in the presence of large amounts of damaged DNA *(142)*. The 14-3-3σ-null cells were very sensitive to killing by adriamycin, probably owing to the catastrophic mitosis. Inactivation of both p21/waf1 and 14-3-3σ in HCT116 led to a severe defect in G2 arrest: such cells were killed much more efficiently by adriamycin than cells lacking either gene alone *(143)*.

7.1. The Role of Transcriptional Repression in G2 Arrest

To understand how the overexpression of p53 could induce G2 arrest, we focused on the regulation of Cdc2, a likely candidate to mediate this effect. In cells arrested in G2 by p53, Cdc2 activity was low, but CAK activity was unaffected *(131)*. Thus, our results suggest that the reduction in threonine 161 phosphorylation of Cdc2 in response to p21/waf1 is not owing to direct inactivation of CAK, and other mechanisms must be at play. Immunoblotting also showed that when cells were just reaching the G2/M boundary (approx 20 h after removal of mimosine), the phosphorylation of Cdc2 at either tyrosine 15 or threonine 14 was not increased by high levels of p53, compared to low levels of p53 *(131)*. However, the level of cyclin B1 was reduced at this time point, and when cells were arrested in G2 for 48 or 72 h, the amount of Cdc2 protein was also downregulated. Loss of both proteins was caused by repression of both promoters by p53 *(131)*. We did not detect 14-3-3σ in these experiments because it appears not to be expressed in fibroblasts. Combining the available data, p53 initially reduces Cdc2 activity by inducing Gadd45, by blocking threonine 161 phosphorylation by way of p21/waf1, and by repressing cyclin B1. Eventually, Cdc2 protein is also downregulated. Interestingly, overexpression of cyclin B1 was sufficient to overcome G2 arrest induced by p53 in an ovarian cancer cell line *(144)*. In our studies, G2 arrest was abrogated

64. Kharbanda, S., Saleem, A., Datta, R., Yuan, Z. M., Weichselbaum, R., and Kufe, D. (1994) Ionizing radiation induces rapid tyrosine phosphorylation of p34cdc2. *Cancer Res.* **54**, 1412–1414.

65. Furnari, B., Rhind, N., and Russell, P. (1997) Cdc25 mitotic inducer targeted by chk1 DNA damage checkpoint kinase [see comments]. *Science* **277**, 1495–1497.

66. Peng, C. Y., Graves, P. R., Thoma, R. S., Wu, Z., Shaw, A. S., and Piwnica-Worms, H. (1997) Mitotic and G2 checkpoint control: regulation of 14-3-3 protein binding by phosphorylation of Cdc25C on serine-216 [see comments]. *Science* **277**, 1501–1505.

67. Sanchez, Y., Wong, C., Thoma, R. S., Richman, R., Wu, Z., Piwnica-Worms, H., and Elledge, S. J. (1997) Conservation of the Chk1 checkpoint pathway in mammals: linkage of DNA damage to Cdk regulation through Cdc25 [see comments]. *Science* **277**, 1497–1501.

68. Walworth, N., Davey, S., and Beach, D. (1993) Fission yeast chk1 protein kinase links the rad checkpoint pathway to cdc2. *Nature* **363**, 368–371.

69. Murakami, H., and Okayama, H. (1995) A kinase from fission yeast responsible for blocking mitosis in S phase. *Nature* **374**, 817–819.

70. McGowan, C. H. (2002) Checking in on Cds1 (Chk2): A checkpoint kinase and tumor suppressor. *Bioessays* **24**, 502–511.

71. Chaturvedi, P., Eng, W. K., Zhu, Y., et al. (1999) Mammalian Chk2 is a downstream effector of the ATM-dependent DNA damage checkpoint pathway. *Oncogene* **18**, 4047–4054.

72. Liu, Q., Guntuku, S., Cui, X. S., et al. (2000) Chk1 is an essential kinase that is regulated by Atr and required for the G(2)/M DNA damage checkpoint. *Genes Dev.* **14**, 1448–1459.

73. Matsuoka, S., Rotman, G., Ogawa, A., Shiloh, Y., Tamai, K., and Elledge, S. J. (2000) Ataxia telangiectasia-mutated phosphorylates chk2 in vivo and in vitro. *Proc. Natl. Acad. Sci. U S A* **97**, 10389–10394.

74. Abraham, R. T. (2001) Cell cycle checkpoint signaling through the ATM and ATR kinases. *Genes Dev.* **15**, 2177–2196.

75. Banin, S., Moyal, L., Shieh, S., et al. (1998) Enhanced phosphorylation of p53 by ATM in response to DNA damage. *Science* **281**, 1674–1677.

76. Canman, C. E., Lim, D. S., Cimprich, K. A., et al. (1998) Activation of the ATM kinase by ionizing radiation and phosphorylation of p53. *Science* **281**, 1677–1679.

77. Siliciano, J. D., Canman, C. E., Taya, Y., Sakaguchi, K., Appella, E., and Kastan, M. B. (1997) DNA damage induces phosphorylation of the amino terminus of p53. *Genes Dev.* **11**, 3471–3481.

78. Cliby, W. A., Roberts, C. J., Cimprich, K. A., et al. (1998) Overexpression of a kinase-inactive ATR protein causes sensitivity to DNA-damaging agents and defects in cell cycle checkpoints. *EMBO J.* **17**, 159–169.

79. Tibbetts, R. S., Brumbaugh, K. M., Williams, J. M., et al. (1999) A role for ATR in the DNA damage-induced phosphorylation of p53. *Genes Dev.* **13**, 152–157.

80. Savitsky, K., Bar-Shira, A., Gilad, S., et al. (1995) A single ataxia telangiectasia gene with a product similar to PI-3 kinase. *Science* **268**, 1749–1753.

81. Bulavin, D. V., Higashimoto, Y., Popoff, I. J., et al. (2001) Initiation of a G2/M checkpoint after ultraviolet radiation requires p38 kinase. *Nature* **411,** 102–107.
82. Baber-Furnari, B. A., Rhind, N., Boddy, M. N., Shanahan, P., Lopez-Girona, A., and Russell, P. (2000) Regulation of mitotic inhibitor Mik1 helps to enforce the DNA damage checkpoint. *Mol. Biol. Cell* **11,** 1–11.
83. Smits, V. A., Klompmaker, R., Arnaud, L., Rijksen, G., Nigg, E. A., and Medema, R. H. (2000) Polo-like kinase-1 is a target of the DNA damage checkpoint. *Nat. Cell Biol.* **2,** 672–676.
84. Griffiths, D. J., Barbet, N. C., McCready, S., Lehmann, A. R., and Carr, A. M. (1995) Fission yeast rad17: a homolog of budding yeast RAD24 that shares regions of sequence similarity with DNA polymerase accessory proteins. *EMBO J.* **14,** 5812–5823.
85. Green, C. M., Erdjument-Bromage, H., Tempst, P., and Lowndes, N. F. (2000) A novel Rad24 checkpoint protein complex closely related to replication factor C.[erratum appears in Curr Biol 2000;10(4):R171]. *Curr. Biol.* **10,** 39–42.
86. St Onge, R. P., Udell, C. M., Casselman, R., and Davey, S. (1999) The human G2 checkpoint control protein hRAD9 is a nuclear phosphoprotein that forms complexes with hRAD1 and hHUS1. *Mol. Biol. Cell* **10,** 1985–1995.
87. Lindsey-Boltz, L. A., Bermudez, V. P., Hurwitz, J., and Sancar, A. (2001) Purification and characterization of human DNA damage checkpoint Rad complexes. *Proc. Natl. Acad. Sci. U S A* **98,** 11236–11241.
88. Venclovas, C., and Thelen, M. P. (2000) Structure-based predictions of Rad1, Rad9, Hus1 and Rad17 participation in sliding clamp and clamp-loading complexes. *Nucleic Acids Res.* **28,** 2481–2493.
89. Walworth, N. C., and Bernards, R. (1996) rad-dependent response of the chk1-encoded protein kinase at the DNA damage checkpoint. *Science* **271,** 353–356.
90. Parker, A. E., Van de Weyer, I., Laus, M. C., Oostveen, I., Yon, J., Verhasselt, P., and Luyten, W. H. (1998) A human homolog of the Schizosaccharomyces pombe rad1+ checkpoint gene encodes an exonuclease. *J. Biol. Chem.* **273,** 18332–18339.
91. Miki, Y., Swensen, J., Shattuck-Eidens, D., et al. (1994) A strong candidate for the breast and ovarian cancer susceptibility gene BRCA1. *Science* **266,** 66–71.
92. Futreal, P. A., Liu, Q., Shattuck-Eidens, D., et al. (1994) BRCA1 mutations in primary breast and ovarian carcinomas. *Science* **266,** 120–122.
93. Scully, R., Chen, J., Ochs, R. L., et al. (1997) Dynamic changes of BRCA1 subnuclear location and phosphorylation state are initiated by DNA damage. *Cell* **90,** 425–435.
94. Wang, Y., Cortez, D., Yazdi, P., Neff, N., Elledge, S. J., and Qin, J. (2000) BASC, a super complex of BRCA1-associated proteins involved in the recognition and repair of aberrant DNA structures. *Genes Dev.* **14,** 927–939.
95. Dolganov, G., Maser, R., Novikov, A., et al. (1996) Human Rad50 is physically associated with human Mre11: identification of a conserved multiprotein complex implicated in recombinational DNA repair. *Mol. Cell. Biol.* **16,** p4832–4841.
96. Maser, R., Monsen, K., Nelms, B., and Petrini, J. (1997) hMre11 and hRad50 nuclear foci are induced during the normal cellular response to DNA double-strand breaks. *Mol. Cell. Biol.* **17,** p6087–6096.

162. Polager, S., and Ginsberg, D. (2003) E2F mediates sustained G2 arrest and down-regulation of Stathmin and AIM-1 expression in response to genotoxic stress. *J. Biol. Chem.* **278**, 1443–1449.

163. Dou, Q. P., Zhao, S., Levin, A. H., Wang, J., Helin, K., and Pardee, A. B. (1994) G1/S-regulated E2F-containing protein complexes bind to the mouse thymidine kinase gene promoter. *J. Biol. Chem.* **269**, 1306–1313.

164. Ishida, S., Huang, E., Zuzan, H., et al. (2001) Role for E2F in control of both DNA replication and mitotic functions as revealed from DNA microarray analysis. *Mol. Cell. Biol.* **21**, 4684–4699.

165. Polager, S., Kalma, Y., Berkovich, E., and Ginsberg, D. (2002) E2Fs up-regulate expression of genes involved in DNA replication, DNA repair and mitosis. *Oncogene* **21**, 437–446.

166. Ren, B., Cam, H., Takahashi, Y., Volkert, T., Terragni, J., Young, R. A., and Dynlacht, B. D. (2002) E2F integrates cell cycle progression with DNA repair, replication, and G(2)/M checkpoints. *Genes Dev.* **16**, 245–256.

167. Chang, B. D., Broude, E. V., Fang, J., V., K. T., Abdryashitov, R., Poole, J. C., and Roninson, I. B. (2000) p21Waf1/Cip1/Sdi1-induced growth arrest is associated with depletion of mitosis-control proteins and leads to abnormal mitosis and endoreduplication in recovering cells. Oncogene 19, 2165–2170.

3

Analyzing the Spindle Checkpoint in Yeast and Frogs

P. Todd Stukenberg and Daniel J. Burke

Summary

The spindle checkpoint is an evolutionarily conserved regulatory mechanism that ensures correct segregation of chromosomes at mitosis and meiosis. The kinetochore plays an integral role in spindle checkpoint signaling by integrating chromosome attachment to the spindle with cell cycle progression. A single kinetochore can inhibit cell cycle progression in the absence of proper spindle attachment or tension from bipolar orientation. Recent advances have shed light on how the kinetochore measures these situations, transduces a signal, and inhibits the entry into anaphase.

Key Words: Spindle; checkpoint; mitosis; regulation, kinetochore; anaphase.

1. Introduction

The original concept of cell cycle checkpoints, formulated by Hartwell and Weinert *(1)*, was developed from the genetic analysis of the budding yeast cell cycle. Hartwell and his students isolated and characterized cell division cycle (cdc) mutants, and their analysis suggested that the cell cycle was organized as a series of precursor–product relationships *(2,3)*. Epistasis experiments suggested a linear order of function for the genes involved in DNA replication and segregation. The model was conceptually simple. DNA replication preceded mitosis because a substrate for mitosis (e.g., centromeres) had to be synthesized during S phase. The precise timing that assured that mitosis did not happen until S phase was complete could be realized if the centromeres were the very last DNA sequences to be replicated. This simple model for how order was achieved in the cell cycle became less tenable as exceptions to the rules accumulated. For example, the mutant *esp1* was so named because mutant cells accumulated multipolar spindles owing to extra spindle pole bodies (the yeast equivalent to centrosomes). Therefore, the mutant cells appeared to uncouple

From: *Methods in Molecular Biology, vol. 280: Checkpoint Controls and Cancer, Volume 1: Reviews and Model Systems*
Edited by: Axel H. Schönthal © Humana Press Inc., Totowa, NJ

spindle assembly from DNA replication *(4)*. It was difficult to reconcile *esp1* with the simple precursor–product model.

Some of the *cdc* mutants appeared to violate their own rules for the precursor–product model of the cell cycle. For example, *cdc17* mutants arrest after S phase, before mitosis *(2)*. However, once the gene was cloned and sequenced, it was shown to be the α-subunit of DNA polymerase *(5)*. *cdc17* mutants should have arrested in early S phase if the precursor–product model were correct. Elegant experiments on the timing of DNA replication in yeast showed that centromeres were among the first sequences to replicate in S phase *(6)*. These and many other observations made it clear that the simple precursor–product model was insufficient to explain how order was achieved in the cell cycle. However, the epistasis experiments were correct and the order of function was as described. So how could the two be reconciled? The answer was both simple and brilliant. The epistasis experiments revealed the order of function but said nothing about the nature of the dependencies. Thus was born the concept of checkpoints. Hartwell and Weinert envisioned a series of regulatory systems (checkpoints) that imposed order on the cell cycle by preventing key transitions from occurring until previous steps were properly completed *(1)*. This chapter focuses on one of them, the spindle checkpoint, which prevents anaphase initiation until all chromosomes are aligned on the mitotic spindle. There are several excellent recent reviews on the spindle checkpoint *(7–11)*. We will outline our current understanding emphasizing the contributions made by genetic analysis of budding yeast and biochemical analysis using *Xenopus* extracts.

2. Experimental Systems

2.1. Yeast

The budding yeast *Saccharomyces cerevisiae* is a model genetic organism that has been invaluable in dissecting the spindle checkpoint. Yeast exists as haploids or diploids and is grown in liquid cultures or on semi-solid media on petri plates. Stable diploids can be isolated and induced to undergo meiosis so that the spindle checkpoint can be analyzed in vegetative and meiotic cells. In addition, meiosis permits a simple method to construct strains of different genotypes. A myriad of molecular tools makes it possible to precisely manipulate genes for a complete molecular analysis of any gene product. Cytological tools are also highly developed, so it is possible to assay the spindle checkpoint in populations of cells as well as in individuals. Chapter 13 provides details for assaying the spindle checkpoint in yeast.

2.2. Xenopus

Upon fertilization, *Xenopus* embryos undergo twelve divisions to generate a blastula of approx 4000 cells. The embryonic cell cycles are very rapid and are devoid of growth phases such that they alternate between S phase and mitosis. To facilitate these rapid divisions, eggs have soluble stockpiles of kinetochore and checkpoint components. Therefore, *Xenopus* extracts are an excellent source to purify kinetochore subassemblies and identify novel kinetochore proteins. Another advantage of *Xenopus* extracts is that kinetochores can be assembled in vitro *(12,13)*. The kinetochores assembled in *Xenopus* egg extracts are functional because they align chromosomes in metaphase *(14)*, segregate chromosomes in anaphase *(15)*, and send spindle checkpoint signals *(13)*. There are in vitro assays for protein localization to *Xenopus* kinetochores as well as kinetochore functions, which allows experimental intervention including immunodepletion of endogenous proteins and replacement with recombinant proteins including mutants.

It is also easy to manipulate the cell cycle state of the extracts. *Xenopus* eggs are naturally arrested in metaphase of meiosis II by cytostatic factor (CSF). Spindles and kinetochores form rapidly when demembranated *Xenopus* sperm are added to mitotic egg extracts (CSF extracts). Adding calcium, which drives mitotic spindles assembled in these extracts to complete anaphase and enter interphase, can then mimic fertilization. The extracts will then replicate chromatin and centrosomes and reenter mitosis with a bipolar spindle. A spindle checkpoint signal is generated in CSF extracts that contain both high levels of sperm nuclei and nocodazole to depolymerize microtubules. These extracts remain in mitosis after calcium addition, unless a component of the spindle checkpoint is inactivated or removed *(13)*. These cell cycle transitions can be easily followed cytologically and biochemically; mitotic extracts in nocodazole contain small condensed chromosomes and high levels of histone H1 kinase activity, whereas interphase extracts have decondensed nuclei and low H1 kinase activity *(16–19)*.

The egg extracts of *Xenopus laevis* perform a number of in vitro reactions that cannot be performed by typical somatic cell lysates. Their uniqueness derives from five main sources. First, extracts are derived from eggs that are naturally arrested in the same cell cycle state, metaphase of meiosis II. Second, eggs are almost 1 µL in vol (thousands of times larger in volume than somatic cells), yet contain only a single genome; therefore, they are almost completely composed of cytoplasm. Third, the eggs are poised to undergo 12 rapid divisions with little protein synthesis; therefore, they have stockpiled almost all the components required for their cell cycles. Fourth, the eggs are full of a dense energy storage granule known as yolk. Gentle centrifugation of the eggs is sufficient to send the dense yolk granules through the plasma membranes to lyse the cells. This cell lysis procedure is extremely gentle, keeping most membrane organelles intact and generating little protein denaturation. Fifth, the extracts are extremely concentrated and contain almost no exogenous buffer. Murray and Kirschner improved the initial egg extracts of Lohka and Masui by adding a "packing spin" containing an oil of intermediate density between buffer and eggs (16). During this spin the round eggs are distorted, pack extremely tightly, and the little space between the eggs is filled with oil rather than buffer. The top layers of buffer and oil are removed and then a 10,000g crushing spin lyses the eggs and generates four layers: a top lipid layer, a thin layer of residual oil, a layer of pure cytosol, and a yolk and pigment granule layer. The intermediate layer, which contains approx 50 mg/mL cytoplasm and many membrane organelles, is used as the extract, and it is a true cytosol derived wholly from egg cytoplasm. However, this cytosol also contains stockpiles of nuclear proteins and nuclear membrane components that are required for the early divisions.

The experimental details to establish spindle checkpoints in *Xenopus* extracts have been previously provided (19,18), and will be expanded in later chapters. Therefore, we will concentrate on the conceptual details of using *Xenopus* extracts here. CSF eggs extracts are generated, and demembranated sperm and nocodazole are added for 30 min to allow the extracts to assemble kinetochores and generate the spindle checkpoint signal. Control extracts do not contain nocodazole. Calcium addition triggers the destruction of CSF and the cell cycle is monitored for an additional hour. Checkpoint competent extracts will remain in mitosis for the entire hour, while extracts that are unable to arrest will exit mitosis within 20 min. The key reagent to address whether a specific protein is required for checkpoint function is a highly specific antibody. Ideally, the antibody will block the function of the protein when added to the extract and will also immunodeplete the protein. The two uses are complementary. In an immunodepletion experiment, one adds back recombinant protein to rescue the effect. The ability to rescue the depleted extract identifies components that are both necessary and sufficient for checkpoint function. The inability to rescue the activity usually suggests that the identified protein is physically associated with other components that are required for checkpoint function. The advantage of adding function-blocking antibodies is that one can preassemble kinetochores, initiate the checkpoint signal, and then block the activity. This has become the standard to address whether a component is required to maintain a preestablished spindle checkpoint signal (20,21).

3. Spindle Checkpoint Genes

3.1. Yeast Genes Identified Through Genetic Approaches

The spindle checkpoint was originally defined in yeast by screens for mutants sensitive to benzimidazole drugs (such as benomyl and nocodazole), which cause microtubules to depolymerize *(22,23)*. Among the sensitive mutants were those that were unable to arrest in mitosis. Two nonoverlapping sets of mutants were identified and named *mad1*, *mad2*, *mad3* (mitotic arrest deficient), and *bub1*, *bub2*, and *bub3* (budding uninhibited by benzimidazoles). Later analysis of a mutant that affected spindle pole duplication and formed monopolar spindles, *mps1*, showed that it had a dual function that included the spindle checkpoint *(24)*.

Two later studies independently identified Cdc55, the B-type regulatory subunit of phosphatase 2A, as a component of the spindle checkpoint that was linked to Cdc28 regulation through inhibitory phosphorylation *(25,26)*. It was shown that Cdc55 regulates the metaphase to anaphase transition in nocodazole-arrested cells, in one of the first uses of GFP-tagged chromosomes in yeast *(25)*. A candidate gene approach identified BFA1 (Byr four alike, because of the homology to a *Schizosaccharomyces pombe* gene), which encodes one member of a two-component GTPase activating protein along with Bub2 *(27,28)*. In addition, the *ipl1* mutants (increase in ploidy) have abrogated checkpoints under certain conditions. The data for *ipl1* are confusing because the mutants arrest in response to nocodazole, which is not expected for a spindle checkpoint mutant. However, the *ipl1* mutant fails to arrest in response to excess expression of Mps1, which activates the spindle checkpoint *(29)*. Further work is needed to clarify the role of Ipl1 in the spindle checkpoint. Finally, the kinetochore is also required for spindle checkpoint signaling *(20,30)*. There are proteins at the kinetochore that sense proper microtubule attachment and in its absence initiate the signal. How the kinetochore performs these roles is still mysterious, although interesting models have been proposed in the aforementioned reviews of the spindle checkpoint. Are the genetics saturating and have all of the genes been identified? It seems unlikely. The original screens found nonoverlapping sets of genes and were not saturated, as proven by the subsequent identification of new genes by candidate gene approaches. Genes with redundant functions are not identified in standard genetic screens, and there has been no systematic approach to identify spindle checkpoint mutants among essential genes. We suspect that there are new genes to be discovered in the future.

3.2. Homologs of the Yeast Spindle Checkpoint Genes

The spindle checkpoint is evolutionarily conserved from yeast to man *(7–10)*. Homologs of most of the spindle checkpoint genes have been identified in

one must assay kinetochore structure. Kinetochore structure is almost impossible to assay rigorously, as the kinetochore contains over 40 known proteins, and probably many others that have not been identified. It would be a daunting task to assay for the presence of each protein in the kinetochore. As a compromise, it is reasonable to use immunofluorescence to localize a subset of proteins to kinetochores in combination with spindle checkpoint assays. Because the kinetochore appears to be made of soluble subcomplexes (CenpA nucleosome, AuroraB/INCENP/survivin, Ndc80 complex, Rod/Zw10 complex, dynactin, dynein, CENP-F, CENP-E, and the checkpoint proteins) that assemble on kinetochores in mitosis, one should strive to assay the presence of each subassembly. Assaying kinetochore assembly in extracts or cells that contain function-blocking antibodies is further complicated by the fact that it is necessary to determine the localization of components with secondary antibodies that do not cross react. Therefore, it is important to generate a collection of kinetochore and checkpoint antibodies in multiple species. Analysis of the spindle checkpoint in metazoans suggests that the kinetochore requirement is more complex than in yeast. In addition to the Ndc80 complex, the AuroraB/INCENP/survivin and Rod/Zw10 complexes are also required for the checkpoint, independent of their roles in kinetochore assembly *(20,34,41,43)*.

Fluorescence recovery experiments show that checkpoint proteins associate transiently with the kinetochore and cycle through at a very high rate *(44,45)*. Mad2 association with the kinetochore requires Mad1*(12)*. However, Mad3 binding to the fission yeast kinetochore is independent of Mad1 and Mad2, but requires Bub1, Bub3, and Mph1, the Mps1 homolog *(46)*. This suggests that there may be at least two independent binding sites for checkpoint proteins in the kinetochore, and distinct complexes may form.

4. Tension, Occupancy, and the Source of the Signal

What event is measured at the kinetochore? There are two models that have been proposed. The first is that tension across the kinetochores, the result of microtubule binding to opposite spindle poles, is assessed, and cells enter anaphase only when all chromosomes are under tension. The second is kinetochore-microtubule occupancy. This model predicts that there are microtubule binding sites in sister kinetochores that must be stably bound by microtubules, and cells enter anaphase only when all sites are occupied. There are data supporting both models *(38,39,47,48)*. There are some proposals that both mechanisms operate and may even be regulated independently *(29,49)*.

There are mutants in budding yeast that enter mitosis in the absence of DNA replication *(48,50)*. If tension across sister kinetochores were required to initiate anaphase, then these mutants should be permanently arrested in mitosis. There is a slight delay in mitosis that depends on the spindle checkpoint, and this has been interpreted to mean that there is a tension-sensitive mechanism operating during yeast mitosis *(50)*. The data are intriguing, but the interpretation is difficult because yeast kinetochores cannot be visualized and it is impossible to know when all of them are attached to microtubules. Kinetochores that are assembled on unreplicated chromosomes may be different from those on fully replicated chromosomes and may bind microtubules less efficiently. Furthermore, *ipl1* mutants eliminate the delay, which could be further evidence that Ipl1 is required for the spindle checkpoint *(29)*. However, a separate study showed that Ipl1promotes bi-orientation of sister kinetochores by detaching kinetochores from microtubules if they are not under tension *(51,52)*. In the absence of DNA replication, Ipl1 clearly detaches chromosomes *(52)*. If the checkpoint measures microtubule occupancy and not tension, and delays cells when chromosomes are detached, then you would expect a mitotic delay in the DNA-replication mutants, because Ipl1 detaches chromosomes under these conditions and that would activate the checkpoint. Therefore, in the absence of DNA replication, you would predict a mitotic delay that would be dependent on the spindle checkpoint and Ipl1. The mutants that perform mitosis in the absence of DNA replication may not distinguish between tension and microtubule occupancy in the yeast spindle checkpoint.

There are similar conflicting data about the existence of both a tension and occupancy checkpoint in metazoans. Classic experiments have demonstrated a role for tension in the meiosis I of certain insect spermatocytes *(39)*. In mitotic cells that have one misoriented chromosome, such that only one of the sister kinetochores is attached to microtubules, laser ablation of the unattached kinetochore abrogates the spindle checkpoint. This result indicates that the unattached kinetochore is required to initiate the spindle checkpoint signal *(53)*. However, after ablation, the sister kinetochore that was attached could not possibly have been under tension, yet it did not inhibit cell cycle progression. This argues that the absence of tension is not the signal that initiates the checkpoint. Low concentrations of vinblastin can arrest cells without tension between sisters. Under these concentrations, both Bub1 and Bubr1 localize to kinetochores. However, there is no Mad2 staining, which suggests that there are two checkpoint pathways, one responsive to tension and a second measuring occupancy *(49)*. Small-molecule inhibitors of Aurora kinase activity inhibit taxol-dependent checkpoint arrest in human cell lines, but these treated cells have a considerable delay in nocodazole (Taylor, S., and Peters, J. M., personal communication). In contrast, injecting antibodies or RNAi to inhibit the activity of Aurora B eliminates the checkpoint, and cells cannot arrest in the presence of either nocodazole or taxol.

Why do the different treatments produce different results? One possible explanation could be the different actions of the drugs. Nocodazole eliminates all microtubules; therefore, chromosomes lack attachments and tension. Taxol eliminates tension but not microtubule occupancy in the kinetochore *(47)*. One interesting explanation is that Aurora kinase activity is required only for the tension checkpoint and is abrogated by small molecule inhibitors. In this model, Aurora kinase activity would induce the kinetochore to release microtubules and thus indirectly trigger the occupancy checkpoint. Because abrogation of any one protein in the Aurora complex eliminates the inner centromere localization of all other members, the Aurora B complex may be additionally required for an occupancy checkpoint, and both functions of the complex may be eliminated by antibodies and RNAi. Further experiments are needed to distinguish whether there are two branches of checkpoint signaling or whether tension regulates occupancy, which then regulates checkpoint signaling.

5. Transducing the Signal

The function of the spindle checkpoint proteins is to transduce the signal from the kinetochore to inhibit the cell cycle machinery. Two protein kinases, Bub1 and Mps1, are among the spindle checkpoint proteins, and there is a third kinase in *Xenopus* and other eucaryotic cells, Bub1R1 *(54)*. The kinase activity of Bub1 is required for the checkpoint in yeast *(55)*. The Mps1 kinase is essential in yeast and required for the checkpoint in *Xenopus (21)*. Neither the Bub1 nor the Bub1R1 kinase activities are required for the checkpoint in *Xenopus*; however, it is untested whether they have redundant functions. Therefore, some aspect of transducing the signal requires protein kinase activity in yeast and *Xenopus*. Yeast Mad1 is a phosphoprotein that is phosphorylated in response to checkpoint activation, and Mps1 can phosphorylate Mad1 in vitro *(56)*. Excess expression of Mps1 can induce yeast cells to arrest in the absence of apparent spindle damage *(56)*. There is also an allele of BUB1 (BUB1-5) that can also arrest cells, and epistasis experiments suggest that Bub1 and Mps1 act interdependently to cause this arrest *(57)*. This suggests that activating the protein kinases could be an initiating event in checkpoint signaling. However, excess Mps1 expression can arrest cells independently of kinetochore function and may not reflect the kinetochore-dependent response to checkpoint activation *(11)*. The importance of Mad1 phosphorylation is also unclear. Mad1 is not phosphorylated in *Xenopus* extracts in response to checkpoint activation and is not a substrate for the *Xenopus* Mps1 in vitro *(21)*. Furthermore, Mad1 is not phosphorylated in response to excess Bub1-5 in yeast, suggesting that phosphorylation of Mad1 is not required for mitotic inhibition *(57)*. The role of the protein kinases and phosphorylation in the spindle checkpoint remains mysterious and is an important area of future research. The in vivo substrates for the kinases need to be found and their role in the spindle checkpoint determined.

Recent attention has been focused on novel protein complexes that form in response to checkpoint activation *(9,46,58–61)*. There are at least three different constitutive complexes of the spindle checkpoint proteins *(62)*. One contains Mad1 and Mad2, another contains Bub1 and Bub3, and a third contains Mad3 (BubR1) and Bub3. Upon checkpoint activation, there are new complexes that form. In both yeast and *Xenopus*, a Mad2–Bub3–Mad3 (BubR1) complex forms, and in yeast a Mad1–Bub1–Bub3 complex forms. The ultimate goal of the kinetochore-activated spindle checkpoint is to prevent sister chromatid separation. Mcd1/Scc1 is a cohesin subunit that aids in holding sister chromatids together and is the substrate of a protease called *separase*, encoded by the ESP1 gene in yeast. Pds1 is the anaphase inhibitor (called *securin*) that regulates the activity of separase. Therefore, restraining the onset of anaphase requires regulating securin. Pds1 is a substrate of the APC/C and is targeted for proteolysis by the specificity factor Cdc20. To inhibit anaphase onset is to prevent Cdc20-dependent proteolysis of securin. This could be accomplished if the spindle checkpoint proteins, in response to checkpoint activation, were inhibitors of Cdc20.

6. Inhibiting the Cell Cycle

Genetic experiments in yeast suggest that Cdc20 is the ultimate target of the spindle checkpoint. Mutations in Cdc20 cause a dominant resistance to checkpoint activation, suggesting that Cdc20 is the effector in the pathway. The mutations map to a small domain that was later shown to be present in both Mad1 and Cdc20. Peptides corresponding to that domain are capable of binding to Mad2 *(60,63)*. There is a conformational change in Mad2 that accompanies binding to the peptide that has led to a model where Mad2 is exchanged from a complex with Mad1 to a complex with Cdc20, with the consequence that Cdc20 is inhibited for Pds1 destruction *(8,60,63)*. What is the role of the kinetochore in the generation of this Mad2–Cdc20 complex? Mad2 localizes to kinetochores during prometatphase and in nocodazole treated cells, and the localization is Mad1 dependent *(12)*. Similarly, Cdc20 associates with kinetochores, and both Mad2 and Cdc20 association with the kinetochore are transient, with half-lives less than 25 s *(45)*. Both proteins rapidly cycle through the kinetochore, and this could explain how kinetochores catalyze the inhibition of Cdc20. There are two models to explain the inhibition. One is that Cdc20 is bound in some complex that sequesters it from the APC/C, and the other is that there is an inhibitor that binds to Cdc20 and directly inhibits the APC/C. Genetic experiments in yeast clearly show that all of the checkpoint genes have a role in inhibiting the cell cycle in response to checkpoint activation, and any biochemical model must explain these dependencies. Experiments using recombinant Mad2 and *Xenopus* extracts support the direct inhibition model and suggest that the inhibitor of Cdc20 is a tetrameric form of Mad2 that binds to a Cdc20–APC/C complex and inhibits the activity *(59)*. However, high concentrations of the tetramer are required for inhibition. Bub1R1 (Mad3 in yeast) is a potent inhibitor of Cdc20 in vitro and can bind to and inhibit Cdc20 and the APC/C *(58)*. Bub1R1 is also purified in an inhibitory complex with stoichiometric amounts of Bub3, Mad2, and Cdc20, named the *mitotic checkpoint complex,* or MCC *(64,65)*. This is a potent inhibitor of the APC/C that forms in both yeast and *Xenopus* in response to checkpoint activation *(61,64)*. Surprisingly, MCC complex formation in yeast occurs in an *ndc10-1* mutant that eliminates kinetochore function, suggesting that this is not the inhibitor that is formed in a kinetochore-dependent manner *(66)*. The complex is constitutive in somatic cells, but made in response to checkpoint signaling in *Xenopus* extracts *(42,65)*. How MCC regulates APC is a critical unanswered question. The sequestering and direct inhibition models are not mutually exclusive. Multiple inhibitors may form in response to different signals, such as the lack of tension or the lack of occupancy, and different pools of Cdc20 and the APC/C may exist.

7. Conclusions

We are beginning to understand certain molecular details of how the spindle checkpoint functions in organisms as diverse as yeast and *Xenopus*. The kinetochore plays an important role in generating the signal and perhaps in the formation of the protein complexes that transduce the signal. We are beginning to understand more about APC/C inhibition. Despite these recent advances, there is much more that is left unanswered. We anticipate that the next few years will be an important time in spindle checkpoint research and that the discoveries will be as exciting as they are illuminating. We also anticipate that both model organisms, yeast and *Xenopus*, will continue to contribute significantly to our understanding of this important cell cycle checkpoint.

References

1. Hartwell, L. H. and Weinert, T. A. (1989) Checkpoints: controls that ensure the order of cell cycle events. *Science* **246,** 629–634.
2. Hartwell, L. H. (1976) Sequential function of gene products relative to DNA synthesis in the yeast cell cycle. *J. Mol. Biol.* **104,** 803–817.
3. Hartwell, L. H., Culotti, J., Pringle, J. R., and Reid, B. J. (1974) Genetic control of the cell division cycle in yeast. *Science* **183,** 46–51.
4. Baum, P., Yip, C., Goetsch, L., and Byers, B. (1988) A yeast gene essential for regulation of spindle pole duplication. *Mol. Cell Biol.* **8,** 5386–5397.
5. Lucchini, G., Falconi, M. M., Pizzagalli, A., Aguilera, A., Klein, H. L., and Plevani, P. (1990) Nucleotide sequence and characterization of temperature-sensitive pol1 mutants of *Saccharomyces cerevisiae. Gene* **90,** 99–104.

6. McCarroll, R. M. and Fangman, W. L. (1988) Time of replication of yeast centromeres and telomeres. *Cell* **54,** 505–513.

7. Burke, D. J. (2000) Complexity in the spindle checkpoint. *Curr. Opin. Genet. Dev.* **10,** 26–31.

8. Musacchio, A. and Hardwick, K. G. (2002) The spindle checkpoint: structural insights into dynamic signalling. *Nat. Rev. Mol. Cell Biol.* **3,** 731–741.

9. Yu, H. (2002) Regulation of APC-Cdc20 by the spindle checkpoint. *Curr. Opin. Cell Biol.* **14,** 706–714.

10. Cleveland, D. W., Mao, Y., and Sullivan, K. F. (2003) Centromeres and kinetochores. From epigenetics to mitotic checkpoint signaling. *Cell* **112,** 407–421.

11. Fraschini, R., Beretta, A., Lucchini, G., and Piatti, S. (2001) Role of the kinetochore protein Ndc10 in mitotic checkpoint activation in *Saccharomyces cerevisiae*. *Mol. Genet. Genomics* **266,** 115–125.

12. Chen, R. H., Shevchenko, A., Mann, M., and Murray, A. W. (1998) Spindle checkpoint protein Xmad1 recruits Xmad2 to unattached kinetochores. *J. Cell Biol.* **143,** 283–295.

13. Minshull, J., Sun, H., Tonks, N. K., and Murray, A. W. (1994) A MAP kinase-dependent spindle assembly checkpoint in *Xenopus* egg extracts. *Cell* **79,** 475–486.

14. Rieder, C. L., Khodjakov, A., Paliulis, L. V., Fortier, T. M., Cole, R. W., and Sluder, G. (1997) Mitosis in vertebrate somatic cells with two spindles: implications for the metaphase/anaphase transition checkpoint and cleavage. *Proc. Natl. Acad. Sci. USA* **94,** 5107–5112.

15. Shamu, C. E. and Murray, A. W. (1992) Sister chromatid separation in frog egg extracts requires DNA topoisomerase II activity during anaphase. *J. Cell Biol.* **117,** 921–934.

16. Murray, A. W. and Kirschner, M. W. (1989) Cyclin synthesis drives the early embryonic cell cycle. *Nature* **339,** 275–280.

17. Murray, A. W., Solomon, M. J., and Kirschner, M. W. (1989) The role of cyclin synthesis and degradation in the control of maturation promoting factor activity. *Nature* **339,** 280–286.

18. Desai, A., Murray, A., Mitchison, T. J., and Walczak, C. E. (1999) The use of *Xenopus* egg extracts to study mitotic spindle assembly and function in vitro. *Methods Cell Biol.* **61,** 385–412.

19. Chen, R. H. and Murray, A. (1997) Characterization of spindle assembly checkpoint in *Xenopus* egg extracts. *Methods Enzymol.* **283,** 572–584.

20. McCleland, M. L., Gardner, R. D., Kallio, M. J., et al. (2003) The highly conserved Ndc80 complex is required for kinetochore assembly, chromosome congression, and spindle checkpoint activity. *Genes Dev.* **17,** 101–114.

21. Abrieu, A., Magnaghi-Jaulin, L., Kahana, J. A., et al. (2001) Mps1 is a kinetochore-associated kinase essential for the vertebrate mitotic checkpoint. *Cell* **106,** 83–93.

22. Li, R. and Murray, A. W. (1991) Feedback control of mitosis in budding yeast. *Cell* **66,** 519–531.

23. Hoyt, M. A., Totis, L., and Roberts, B. T. (1991) *S. cerevisiae* genes required for cell cycle arrest in response to loss of microtubule function. *Cell* **66,** 507–517.

24. Weiss, E. and Winey, M. (1996) The *Saccharomyces cerevisiae* spindle pole body duplication gene MPS1 is part of a mitotic checkpoint. *J. Cell Biol.* **132,** 111–123.

25. Minshull, J., Straight, A., Rudner, A. D., Dernburg, A. F., Belmont, A., and Murray, A. W. (1996) Protein phosphatase 2A regulates MPF activity and sister chromatid cohesion in budding yeast. *Curr. Biol.* **6,** 1609–1620.

26. Wang, Y. and Burke, D. J. (1996) A B-type regulatory subunit of PP2A has multiple roles in mitosis and is required for the kinetochore spindle checkpoint in *Saccharomyces cerevisiae. Mol. Cell. Biol.* **17,** 620–626.

27. Alexandru, G., Zachariae, W., Schleiffer, A., and Nasmyth, K. (1999) Sister chromatid separation and chromosome re-duplication are regulated by different mechanisms in response to spindle damage. *EMBO J.* **18,** 2707–2721.

28. Li, R. (1999) Bifurcation of the mitotic checkpoint pathway in budding yeast. *Proc. Natl. Acad. Sci. USA* **96,** 4989–4994.

29. Biggins, S. and Murray, A. W. (2001) The budding yeast protein kinase Ipl1/Aurora allows the absence of tension to activate the spindle checkpoint. *Genes Dev.* **15,** 3118–3129.

30. Gardner, R. D., Poddar, A., Yellman, C., Tavormina, P. A., Monteagudo, M. C., and Burke, D. J. (2001) The spindle checkpoint of the yeast *Saccharomyces cerevisiae* requires kinetochore function and maps to the CBF3 domain. *Genetics* **157,** 1493–1502.

31. Li, Y. and Benezra, R. (1996) Identification of a human mitotic checkpoint gene: hsMAD2. *Science* **274,** 246–248.

32. Taylor, S. S., Ha, E., and McKeon, F. (1998) The human homologue of Bub3 is required for kinetochore localization of Bub1 and a Mad3/Bub1-related protein kinase. *J. Cell Biol.* **142,** 1–11.

33. Taylor, S. S. and McKeon, F. (1997) Kinetochore localization of murine Bub1 is required for normal mitotic timing and checkpoint response to spindle damage. *Cell* **89,** 727–735.

34. Kallio, M. J., McCleland, M. L., Stukenberg, P. T., and Gorbsky, G. J. (2002) Inhibition of Aurora B kinase blocks chromosome segregation, overrides the spindle checkpoint, and perturbs microtubule dynamics in mitosis. *Curr. Biol.* **12,** 900–905.

35. Cid, V. J., Jimenez, J., Molina, M., Sanchez, M., Nombela, C., and Thorner, J. W. (2002) Orchestrating the cell cycle in yeast: sequential localization of key mitotic regulators at the spindle pole and the bud neck. *Microbiology* **148,** 2647–2659.

36. Cheeseman, I. M., Drubin, D. G., and Barnes, G. (2002) Simple centromere, complex kinetochore: linking spindle microtubules and centromeric DNA in budding yeast. *J. Cell Biol.* **157,** 199–203.

37. Spencer, F. and Hieter, P. (1992) Centromere DNA mutations induce a mitotic delay in *Saccharomyces cerevisiae. Proc. Natl. Acad. Sci. USA* **89,** 8908–8912.

38. Nicklas, R. B. (1997) How cells get the right chromosomes. *Science* **275,** 632–637.

39. Li, X. and Nicklas, R. B. (1995) Mitotic forces control a cell-cycle checkpoint. *Nature* **373,** 630–632.

40. Dohmen, R. J., Wu, P., and Varshavsky, A. (1994) Heat-inducible degron: a method for constructing temperature-sensitive mutants. *Science* **263,** 1273–1276.

41. Chan, G. K., Jablonski, S. A., Starr, D. A., Goldberg, M. L., and Yen, T. J. (2000) Human Zw10 and ROD are mitotic checkpoint proteins that bind to kinetochores. *Nat. Cell Biol.* **2,** 944–947.

42. Chen, R. H. (2002) BubR1 is essential for kinetochore localization of other spindle checkpoint proteins and its phosphorylation requires Mad1. *J. Cell Biol.* **158,** 487–496.

43. Basto, R., Gomes, R., and Karess, R. E. (2000) Rough deal and Zw10 are required for the metaphase checkpoint in *Drosophila. Nat. Cell Biol.* **2,** 939–943.

44. Howell, B. J., Hoffman, D. B., Fang, G., Murray, A. W., and Salmon, E. D. (2000) Visualization of Mad2 dynamics at kinetochores, along spindle fibers, and at spindle poles in living cells. *J. Cell Biol.* **150,** 1233–1250.

45. Kallio, M. J., Beardmore, V. A., Weinstein, J., and Gorbsky, G. J. (2002) Rapid microtubule-independent dynamics of Cdc20 at kinetochores and centrosomes in mammalian cells. *J. Cell Biol.* **158,** 841–847.

46. Millband, D. N. and Hardwick, K. G. (2002) Fission yeast Mad3p is required for Mad2p to inhibit the anaphase-promoting complex and localizes to kinetochores in a Bub1p-, Bub3p-, and Mph1p-dependent manner. *Mol. Cell Biol.* **22,** 2728–2742.

47. Waters, J. C., Chen, R. H., Murray, A. W., and Salmon, E. D. (1998) Localization of Mad2 to kinetochores depends on microtubule attachment, not tension. *J. Cell Biol.* **141,** 1181–1191.

48. Stern, B. M. and Murray, A. W. (2001) Lack of tension at kinetochores activates the spindle checkpoint in budding yeast. *Curr. Biol.* **11,** 1462–1467.

49. Skoufias, D. A., Andreassen, P. R., Lacroix, F. B., Wilson, L., and Margolis, R. L. (2001) Mammalian mad2 and bub1/bubR1 recognize distinct spindle-attachment and kinetochore-tension checkpoints. *Proc. Natl. Acad. Sci. USA* **98,** 4492–4497.

50. Piatti, S., Lengauer, C., and Nasmyth, K. (1995) Cdc6 is an unstable protein whose *de novo* synthesis in G1 is important for the onset of S phase and for preventing a 'reductional' anaphase in the budding yeast *Saccharomyces cerevisiae. EMBO J.* **14,** 3788–3799.

51. Tanaka, T. U. (2002) Bi-orienting chromosomes on the mitotic spindle. *Curr. Opin. Cell Biol.* **14,** 365–371.

52. Tanaka, T. U., Rachidi, N., Janke, C., et al. (2002) Evidence that the Ipl1–Sli15 (Aurora kinase–INCENP) complex promotes chromosome bi-orientation by altering kinetochore-spindle pole connections. *Cell* **108,** 317–329.

53. Rieder, C. L., Cole, R. W., Khodjakov, A., and Sluder, G. (1995) The checkpoint delaying anaphase in response to chromosome monoorientation is mediated by an inhibitory signal produced by unattached kinetochores. *J. Cell Biol.* **130,** 941–948.

54. Chan, G. K., Jablonski, S. A., Sudakin, V., Hittle, J. C., and Yen, T. J. (1999) Human BUBR1 is a mitotic checkpoint kinase that monitors CENP-E functions at kinetochores and binds the cyclosome/APC. *J. Cell Biol.* **146,** 941–954.

55. Roberts, B. T., Farr, K. A., and Hoyt, M. A. (1994) The *Saccharomyces cerevisiae* checkpoint gene BUB1 encodes a novel protein kinase. *Mol. Cell Biol.* **14,** 8282–8291.

Table 1. Cell Cycle-Specific Cyclin/Cdk Complexes, Regulators, and Substrates

Cell cycle Phase	Active cyclin/Cdk complexes	Inhibitors	Activators	Substrates
G1	cyclinD/Cdk4/6	INK4 family	CIP/KIP cdc25A, CAK	Rb
G1/S	cyclin E/Cdk2	WAF1/KIP1	cdc25A	Rb, MCM, cyclin E, Cdc6, Mps1p, Nucleophosmin, NPAT
S	cyclin A/ Cdk2	p21 CKI family	cdc25, CAK	pre-RC Cdt1/ Cdc45
G2	cyclin A/Cdk1	p21 CKI family	cdc25, CAK	E2F1
G2/M	cyclin B/Cdk1	p21 CKI family	cdc25, CAK	MAP4, Eg5. H1-H3 histones Lamins. Securin Integral membrane Proteins, cdc25C

tion of the previous one. Once cells divide into two daughter cells, the cells need some time to again become active and ready to divide, before entering the G1 phase. This is sometimes called G0, or the quiescent phase. Although there is no gene identified so far that encodes a checkpoint protein in G0 phase for the cells to create an environment for the next cell division, the cells must reach the homeostatic size, and in metazoans the cellular size. This depends on the cellular nutrients and both external and internal mitotic stimuli. Cell growth and cell division are sometimes misunderstood, but in real terms cell growth is measured by the cell size and the protein mass. However, in certain cell types such as neurons, oocytes, or muscle cells, cell growth might take place without cell division, whereas in fertilized eggs, cell division may occur without an increase in cell mass. Thus, if cell divison occurs without the cell mass increase, there will be a decrease in the cell size, causing deleterious effects on normal cell divison. Thus, for division to occur, cells must reach sufficient cell mass for the daughter cells before divison gets started. Ribosome biosynthesis is one of the key processes before a cell is ready to divide *(99)*. The S6 kinase phosphorylates the ribosomal protein to accomplish this through the insulin receptor pathways, including PI3K/PDK1 *(100,101)* (**Fig. 1**). TOR, a member of the PI3 kinase family, also regulates the S6 kinase, which maintains actin organization, transcription, and ribosomal biosynthesis. TOR also affects trans-

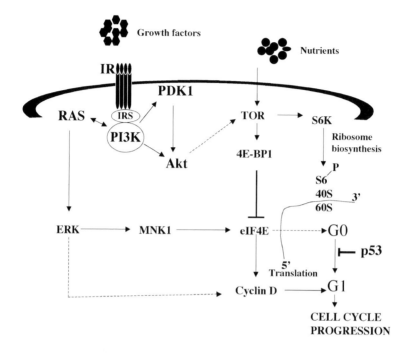

Fig. 1. G0/G1 cell cycle progression and quiescent checkpoint. Ribosome biosynthesis machinery can be activated and deactivated by Ras/PI3K-AKT-TOR-S6K owing to the availability of nutrients and growth factors. Modification of p53 also regulates the quiescent checkpoint. Ras also can activate ERK/MNK1 kinase activity and result in protein synthesis. The RAS/ERK cascade is also known to signal cyclin D-p27 to induce progression through G1.

lation of cyclin D and Myc by phosphorylating 4E-Bp1 (a translational inhibitor also target by Akt). This causes dissociation from the initiation factor eIEF4E. ERK, the mitogen-activated protein kinase, phosphorylates MNK1, which in turn phosphorylates eIEF4E *(102,103)*. The RAS/ERK cascade also regulates cyclin D or KIP1 to allow progression through G1 *(104)*. p27 levels are high and maintain an arrested state in quiescent cells. However, once the cells are exposed to mitogens, p27 gets phosphorylated and subsequently degraded by the proteosome system *(105)*. Similarly, acetylation or Ser-15 phosphorylation of p53 increases in human fibroblasts undergoing replicative senescence or Ras-induced premature senescence, suggesting p53 might have some role in the senescence checkpoint *(106)*. Very recently, the role of p300 as a universal checkpoint function in senescent or differentiated cells has been described in a tetracycline-responsive p300 expressing in the Rat-1 cell line. In serum-stimulated cells, p300 is induced, and that causes inhibition of c-Myc

will be easier to move to the opposite pole at anaphase. This occurs by histone deposition on chromatids, with different types of modifications on the histone including acetylation and phosphorylation *(94–97)*. The histones H1 and H3 can be phosphorylated by different kinases, including cyclin B1–Cdk1 and aurora kinases *(90)*. The linker histone generally gets phosphorylated by cyclin B1–Cdk1 and makes it more condensed. Three enzymes activate Cdk1: the phosphatase Cdc25C, and the kinases Wee1 and Myt1. On one hand, Cdc25C is inhibited by Chk1 and Chk2 kinases, but on the other hand, Wee1 and Myt1 are upregulated by the same pathways *(145,146)*. Plk1 also activates Cdc25C and simultaneously downregulates Wee1 and Myt1 *(147,148)*. Recently, the role of *chfr* as a checkpoint gene in the prophase–prometaphase transition has been described, although the mechanism is not known (**Fig. 4**). Absence of the *chfr* gene in cells causes early entrance of the dividing cells into the prometaphase stage as compared to the wild-type cells, suggesting that Chfr might act as a checkpoint protein *(149)*. Similarly, the passenger protein TD-60, an RCC1 family member of guanine nucleotide exchange factors (GEFs) protein, which binds preferentially the nucleotide-free form of the small G protein Rac1, has checkpoint functions (**Fig. 4**). Suppression of TD-60 causes prometaphase arrest of cells, suppresses spindle assembly, and activates the spindle assembly checkpoint, suggesting a role in the prometaphase to metaphase progression *(150)*. TD-60 is associated with the inner centromeres of metaphase chromosomes, is specific to late G2 and mitosis, and migrates to the spindle midzone in anaphase. TD-60 suppression leads to a general inhibition of spindle assembly, suggesting that it may play a global role in mitotic spindle formation and function. Biochemical identification of mitotic chromosome-associated factors led to the discovery of condensin and cohesin. The core of the subunits contains chromosomal ATPases of the structural maintenance of chromosomes (SMC) protein family. However, the two complexes are structurally and functionally different from each other. Mutational analysis with respect to functional consequences in cohesin and condensin subunits shows roles in gene regulation, DNA repair, cell cycle checkpoints, and centromere structure *(151–154)*. Cohesin is a four-member protein complex, which holds together the sister chromatids of newly replicated DNA. It contains a heterodimer of the SMC proteins Smc1 and Smc3 that is associated with the non-SMC proteins Scc1 and Scc3. The cohesin is loaded to the chromatids at replication and dissociated at anaphase in lower organisms *(155,156)*. However, in higher organisms, the bulk of cohesin is released at prophase, and a smaller amount persists until anaphase at the centromeres *(157)*. Dissociation of cohesin at anaphase is triggered by the proteolytic cleavage of Scc1 by the enzyme separase. Separase is inhibited by a protein called securin until the anaphase-promoting complex ubiquitylates and destroys securin *(160)*. However, condensin is a five-member protein complex that is required for chromosome organization and segregation. It contains a heterodimer of SMC proteins (Smc2 and 4) and three associated non-SMC proteins (CAP-D2, CAP-G, and CAP-H). The five-member protein complex was named *condensin* because sperm chromosomes introduced into egg extracts depleted of any subunits form a diffuse mass rather than a condensed structure *(161,162)*. The molecular mechanisms by which cohesin attaches sister chromatids and condensin to cause reconfiguration remain unsolved. However, the mode of action was recently discovered (*154* and references therein). When incubated with relaxed circular DNA in the presence of topoisomerase I, condensin causes ATP-dependent positive supercoiling, while in the presence of type II topoisomerase, condensin coverts nicked circular DNA into positive knots. In contrast, cohesin catenates nicked circular DNA in the presence of topoisomerase II and causes DNA protein aggregates in gel shift experiments. Thus, condensin has intramolecular activities while cohesin has intermolecular activities. Atomic-force microscopy suggests a "loop fastener" model, in which the condensin hinge binds one region of DNA and then the non-SMC proteins mediate an ATP-dependent opening and closing of SMC "V" to enclose the loop of DNA. The electron spectroscopic imaging of condensin suggests an orientated gyre model, where an ATP-hydrolysis cycle changes the conformation of condensin and allows it to trap two orientated positive supercoil arms. The embrace model of cohesin proposes that Smc1 and 3 are linked at one end by hinge interaction and at the other by interaction with Scc1, so that a large loop forms that encircles both sister chromatids fastened by Scc1 at one end, until proteolytic cleavage of Scc1 disrupts the cohesin loop *(154)*. The role of these two proteins in checkpoint control after DNA damage has been discovered, and that is discussed in the **Subheading 9.**

8.2. Spindle Assembly Checkpoint

Genetic studies in yeast as well as laser ablation and micromanipulation studies in animal cells have identified a checkpoint that delays sister-chromatid separation (**Fig. 4**) *(163)*. To ensure equal segregation of each homologous chromosome, the kinetochores in each sister chromatid pair must interact with microtubules, referred to as bipolar attachment. Several mitotic checkpoint proteins, including Mad1, Mad2, Bub1, Bub3, BubR1, Mbs1, and CENP-E have now been shown to be kinetochore-associated and function as regulators of the spindle checkpoint *(90,163,164)*. This checkpoint monitors the attachment of microtubules to the kinetochores and the generation of tension for chromosome movement. This is also called the kinetochore attachment checkpoint. The kinetochores act as a catalytic site for the production of the "wait anaphase signal." In both budding and fission yeast, the checkpoint is an accessory sub-

have some role in a spindle-positioning checkpoint *(214)*. GTPase Ran not only acts as a regulator of nuclear transport, but also plays a role in mitotic spindle assembly *(215)*. Ran regulates the frequency of transition from shrinkage to growth of microtubules, as well as the capacity of centrosomes to nucleate microtubules *(215,216)*. Wild and coworkers suggested the importance of the balance of microtubule motor activities, particularly that of Eg5. Ran-GTP releases some microtubule-associated proteins (MAPs) to participate in spindle assembly *(217)*. Importin-β sequesters MAP-TPX2 and NuMA, which act as the Ran effector for spindle assembly. The interaction of importin-β occurs with the respective MAPs either directly or indirectly through importin-α. During interphase, Ran-GTP dissociates cargo from importins only in the nucleus, conferring directionality to nuclear transport *(218–221)*. However, in mitosis, Ran-GTP interacts with RCC1 (nucleotide exchange factor) around chromatin. Thus Ran-GTP dissociates the spindle assembly effector from importins in a small perimeter around chromatin by acting as a checkpoint protein, thereby ensuring that they build the spindle in the right place *(218–221)*.

8.4. Cytokinesis or C Phase Checkpoint

When cells undergo mitosis, two processes take place: the division of the membrane and cytosol, and the regulated segregation of the centrosomes (spindle pole bodies) and the chromosomes (**Fig. 4**). These two components are essential for cell survival. Suppression of aurora and IpI1-like midbody-associated protein (AIM-1) kinase activity by dominant negative AIM-1 disrupts cleavage furrow formation without affecting nuclear division and without cytokinesis and subsequent cell death, suggesting that AIM-1 is required for the proper progression of cytokinesis in mammalian cells *(222)*. The Rho family of small GTPases consists of Rho A, Rac, and Cdc42, and regulates many molecular switches of diverse biological function, including remodeling of cytoplasmic actin and microtubules *(223)*. The small GTPase Rho localizes in the cleavage furrow during cytokinesis *(223,225)*. In *Xenopus* eggs, microinjection of either the Rho-specific inhibitor C3, an exoenzyme from *Clostridium botulinum*, or a constitutively active mutant RhoA^{G14V} prevents the progression of cytokinesis, suggesting the importance of Rho in this process *(223)*. Several guanine nucleotide exchange factors (GEFs) are implicated in Rho's activation. One such GEF is ECT2, which co-localizes with the mitotic spindle in metaphase, transfers to the mid-zone in anaphase and telophase, and moves to the midbody in cytokinesis. ECT2 activation depends on its phosphorylation *(226)*. Very recently, the GTPase activating protein (GAP) MgcRacGAP has been reported to co-localize with the mitotic spindle in metaphase, transfer to the mid-zone in anaphase, and accumulate at the midbody in cytokinesis *(227)*.

MgcRacGAP is co-localized with aurora B and RhoA, and not with Rac1/ Cdc42, at the midbody. Aurora B phosphorylates MagRacGAP at Ser 387, and expression of dominant negative aurora B disrupts MgcRacGAP phosphorylation and cytokinesis. Similarly, overexpression of the MagRacGAP S387D mutant arrests cytokinesis at a late stage and induces polyploidy. This provides evidence for the importance of GAP in cytokinesis, along with the involvement of aurora kinase in the regulatory mechanism *(228)*. In addition, polo-like kinases also control mitotic exit by regulating the anaphase-promoting complex, and have been implicated in the temporal and spatial coordination of cytokinesis *(229)*.

9. DNA Damage Checkpoint Genes

The DNA damage checkpoint is a signal cascade that blocks the cell cycle at G1, G2, or metaphase, or slows the rate of DNA replication in S phase. Besides cell cycle blockage, cells respond in different ways, including apoptosis, DNA repair, and activation of transcription. There are many genes involved in DNA damage checkpoint pathways that control both repair and cell cycle progression. However, it is beyond the scope of this article to discuss all their details. The most important genes and their functional regulation will be covered in this section. Once cell DNA is damaged, not only are checkpoints activated, but repair genes are activated at almost the same time. The major DNA damage checkpoint pathways operate in cycling cells. Again, this can be divided into a G1 DNA damage checkpoint, a DNA damage replication or S phase checkpoint, and a G2 DNA damage checkpoint *(230–233)*. On the basis of their positions and functions in the pathways, the checkpoint cascades have been subclassified into DNA damage sensors, signal transducers, and effectors *(234)*. DNA damage checkpoint proteins are well conserved among different organisms, although some differences in the signaling pathways have been identified. A DNA damage checkpoint gene generally performs several functions, including cell cycle delay, activation of DNA repair, maintenance of cell cycle arrest until DNA repair is complete, and reinitiation of cell cycle progression. Activation of checkpoint genes leads to changes in gene expression along with synthesis, degradation, and movement of different proteins.

In mammals, the DNA damage checkpoints can be triggered in any phase of the cell cycle, which may lead to a cell cycle block, DNA repair, or apoptosis. Checkpoint activation is required for cells to arrest in G1, S, and G2 phases, and the substrates include p53, Mdm2, and Chk2 in the G1 checkpoint; Nbs1, Brca1, FancD1, and SMC1 in the transient IR-induced S phase arrest; and Brca1 and hRad17 in the G2/M arrest. A schematic diagram of these pathways is shown in **Figs. 7** and **8**.

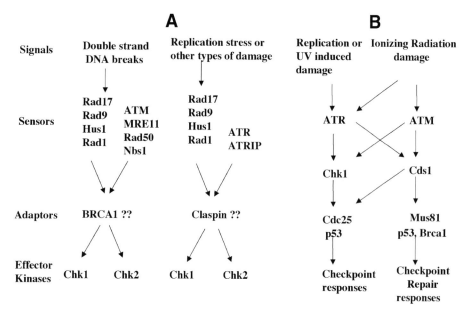

A   **B**

| Signals | Double strand DNA breaks | Replication stress or other types of damage | Replication or UV induced damage | Ionizing Radiation damage |

Fig. 7. DNA damage and replication checkpoint response pathways in eukaryotes. (**A**) Components of a checkpoint signaling pathway arising from the replication block or DNA damage (DSB/SSB) are shown. Rad17–Rad9–Hus1–Rad1 and MRE11–Rad53–Nbs1–ATM complexes can act as sensors after double-strand breaks. Similarly, Rad17–Rad9–Hus1–Rad1 and ATR–ATRIP complexes act after replication or other types of DNA damage. BRCA1/claspin can act as adaptors in the DNA damage response. Chk1/Chk2 act as effector kinases. (**B**) ATR–Chk1 or ATR–Chk2 can be activated after replication stress or UV damage and cause phosphorylation of Cdc25 or p53 for checkpoint responses. However, after ionizing radiation, ATM can activate Chk1/Chk2, which phosphorylate Mus81, p53, or Brca1 to perform checkpoint and repair responses.

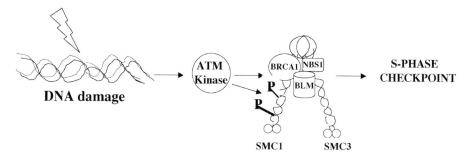

Fig. 8. Cohesin subunits participate in DNA damage checkpoint response. After irradiation, ATM gets activated and phosphorylates the cohesin subunit SMC1. SMC is present in the NBS1, BLM, and Brca1 complexes, and free from cohesin after DNA damage. Phosphorylation of SMC1 is required for the DNA damage S checkpoint.

9.1. ATM-ATR Kinases in the DNA Damage Checkpoint Response

There are many kinases involved in the DNA damage checkpoint pathways. The mammalian members of the ATM family at present include five protein kinases: ATM, ATR, ATX/SMG-1, mTOR/FRAP, DNA-PKcs, and TRRAP *(230–235)*. These kinases are conserved from yeast to mammals and respond to various stresses through phosphorylation of downstream substrates. ATM belongs to a conserved family of proteins having serine/threonine-kinase activity. ATM and DNA-PK respond to double-strand breaks (DSBs), while ATR and ATX respond to both UV light damage and DSBs. Simultaneously, ATR also responds to DNA methylation by methyl methane sulfonate (MMS) and stalled replication forks by replication inhibitors such as hydroxyurea and aphidicolin. mTOR/FRAP responds to nutrient levels and mitogenic stimuli contributing to protein translation, degradation, and growth, but does not have a role in DNA-damage pathways *(233,235)*.

The *ATM* gene encodes a 370-kDa protein. The 350-amino-acid carboxy terminus contains the kinase domain. Exposure of cells to IR triggers ATM kinase activity, leading to phosphorylation of different substrates. The signals sensed by ATM and ATR are transmitted through two effector kinases, Cds1 and Chk1 *(230–235)*. These two effector kinases are conserved in eukaryotes. However, the functional aspects of these kinases are different in lower eukaryotes. In the fission yeast *S. pombe*, Cds1 is the effector of the replication checkpoint and Chk1 is the effector of the G2 DNA damage checkpoint, and it does not respond to incompletely replicated DNA. However, in *S. cerevisiae*, the Cds1 homolog Rad53 functions as both replication and DNA damage checkpoint protein. Chk1 acts at a G2 DNA damage checkpoint in parallel with Rad53 *(230)*.

ATR is associated with Rad26 and is recruited to DNA damage sites *(231,237–239)*. Deletion of human or yeast Rad26 from cells makes ATR functionless. In contrast, deletion of *S. cerevisiae* Ddc2 (Rad26) has no effect on ATR function in vitro. Although ATR phosphorylates Rad26, the significance of this phosphorylation is not known. However, ATR activities increase after Rad26 phosphorylation. Using chromatin immunoprecipitation and GFP fusion protein localization, it has been shown that Ddc2 (Rad26) and Mec1 (ATR) localize to double-stranded DNA breaks in vivo in *S. cerevisiae* *(239)*. However, recruitment of Ddc2 (Rad26) requires Mec1 (ATR), as absence of the latter does not allow recruitment of Rad26 efficiently to the break sites *(240)*. Thus, ATR needs an accessory protein for its recruitment to damage sites on DNA and for its subsequent activation.

ATM may associate with damaged DNA *(241–243)*. A model has been proposed for ATM/ATR activation involving autophosphorylation following DNA damage. ATM molecules are in dimer or multimer and blocked by the FAT domain in an inactive configuration in undamaged cells. Following DNA damage, each ATM molecule phosphorylates another on serine 1981 within the FAT domain, releases the two molecules from each other, and becomes active *(243).* ATM can be found both in the nucleoplasm or bound to the chromatin of DSBs, revealing that ATM phosphorylates not only substrates bound to a DSB site but also substrates in the nucleoplasm before it can load onto the chromatin for DNA repair. hATM does not phosphorylate hATRIP (Rad26) in vitro *(238).* On the other hand, hNbs1 present in the Rad50–Mre11–Nbs1 complex appears to be involved in repair and processing of DNA breaks, and gets phosphorylated by ATM *(245).* Mutations in hATM or hNbs1 cause similar cancer-prone syndromes. ATM phosphorylates different sites on NBS1, including Ser 343 and Ser 278 *(246,247).* Similarly Tel1 (ATM) in *S. cerevisiae* also phosphorylates Xrs2 (Nbs1), and the function of Tel1 is detectable only in Mec1 (ATR) deleted cells *(248,249).* Tel1 also maintains telomere length associated with the Rad50 complex, demonstrating that ATM is dependent on the Rad50–Nbs1–Mre11 complex for its DNA repair and checkpoint effects *(250).*

Comparison of the action of ATM and ATR demonstrates that ATM activation is the initial and most rapid phase of the damage response and is complete within 1–2 h. However, ATR is recruited later and maintains the phosphorylated states of specific substrates. Besides the late activation in some break types, ATR also takes care of specific DNA damage such as UV, stalled replication forks, and hypoxia by phosphorylating specific substrates such as p53 and BRCA1 *(251,252).* Thus, although ATM is the first to respond to DSBs, loss or mutation of ATM does not lead to cell death, while ATR loss leads to both embryonic lethality in mice and loss of viability in cell culture. The significance of ATR is further supported by a study where loss of ATR caused an increase in the fragility of chromosomes, but this was not observed in ATM-deficient cells *(230–234,253).*

9.2. Checkpoint Signaling Through Chk1 and Chk2, the Downstream Target of ATM/ATR/ATX

Chk1 and Chk2 regulate basic cellular functions such as DNA replication and cell-cycle progression, chromatin restructuring, and apoptosis *(230–234).* Structurally unrelated but functionally related serine/threonine kinases Chk1/Chk2 are activated in response to DNA damage. Chk2 is a stable protein expressed throughout the cell cycle, and activated after double-strand breaks by ATM *(254–256).* However, Chk1 is labile, S/G2-specific, activated in unperturbed cells, and also activated by both replication block or DNA damage, and mainly acts through the kinase ATR *(255,256).* Recent reports suggest that the crosstalk between these kinases makes them more flexible in their kinase action *(257,258)*. Thus ATM also can phosphorylate Chk1 by IR that phosphorylates Tlk kinases and causes chromatin remodeling in response to various stresses. Similarly, ATM-independent activation of Chk2 has also been reported *(259)*. In addition, the BRCT repeat, containing proteins including 53BP1, BRCA1, and MDC1, can act as mediators of checkpoint responses *(256,260,261)*. Chk1 and Chk2 kinases phosphorylate Tlk kinase, PML protein, PLK3 kinase, or the E2F1 transcription factors, including the known substrates such as p53, BRCA1, Cdc25C, Cdc25A, and so on *(230–234,262–266)*. Live-cell imaging of Chk2 in mice revealed a distribution of the protein throughout the cells, not localized in foci, suggesting the action of Chk2 as a checkpoint signal spreader *(267)*.

Results from the knockout of Chk1 and Chk2 in mice indicate that Chk1 is essential for mammalian development and viability *(268,269)*, whereas Chk2 is not required *(270,271)*. Despite early embryonic lethality of Chk1-deficient mice, and also lethality of embryonic cells, some important observations reveal that Chk1 has a checkpoint function in the S/M and G2/M transitions *(272)*. Similarly, RNAi-mediated knockout of Chk1 also suggests that it has a role in Cdc25A stabilization in both normal S phase and the intra-S-phase DNA-damage checkpoint in mammalian cells *(273,274)*. A Chk1 requirement in the G2/M checkpoint in response to IR or genotoxic agents has also been reported. However, Chk2-deficient mice are viable, fertile, and not tumor prone *(270,271)*. Dfp1 is one of the targets of Chk2; along with Hsk1, it phosphorylates the substrates of replication origins once there is DNA damage or replication stress, resulting in blockage at the activation of replication origins *(275)*. Similar processes were also proposed in budding yeast, in Rad53-dependent late-firing replication origins *(276)*. However, in *S. pombe*, Cds1 is necessary for survival in S phase after arrest but not for mitotic delay *(277)*.

9.3. 9-1-1 Complexes in Checkpoint Initiation

PCNA forms a homo-trimer that acts as a processivity factor by interacting with DNA polymerase delta at DNA replication sites. The 9-1-1 (Rad9–Rad1–Hus1) complexes have sequence similarity with PCNA and are present in damaged and undamaged cells, indicating they have a role not only in DNA repair but probably also in normal replication pathways *(278)*. Deletions of these 9-1-1 genes have similar checkpoint and damage sensitivity effects in *S. pombe* or *S. cerevisiae*. However, in human cells, the 9-1-1 complex associates with chromatin after DNA damage, whereas in *S. cerevisiae* it localizes to the double-strand breaks and depends on the Rad1, Hus1, and Rad24 (Rad17) proteins *(279–281)*. Rad17 is similar in sequence to replication factor C (RFC) 1. RFC consists of five subunits, recognizes the primer-template junction, and functions to open the PCNA complex for loading onto DNA. *S. cerevisiae* Rad24

(Rad17) replaces RFC1 and binds with the other four subunits of RFC. Bacterial RFC-1 (called δ) forms a stable complex with the PCNA homolog (called β) *(282)*. ATM and ATR phosphorylate Rad17 on two serine residues and regulate the G1-S and G2-M transitions *(283,284)*. Depletion of Rad17 by siRNA also reduces the damage-induced chromatin association of hRad9. Thus, 9-1-1 complexes are loaded onto damaged DNA by the Rad17–RFC complex *(285,286)*. After DNA damage, the PCNA/RFC complex (Rad9, Hus1, Rad1, and Rad17) is phosphorylated in yeast and mammals *(282–284,287,288)*. Constitutively phosphorylated hRad9 gets hyperphosphorylated by ATM after exposure to IR *(288)*. Phosphorylation of serine residues in hRad9 and hRad17 produced checkpoint-deficient alleles *(283,284,288)*. However, phosphorylation is not important for their association, as without DNA damage there is still complex formation *(281)*. Similar findings have been reported in yeast for Ddc1 (Rad9), which requires ATR for phosphorylation and loading onto DSBs *(289,290)*. These studies also suggest that Rad24 (Rad17) does not require Mec1 (ATR) or Tel1 to load Ddc1 (Rad9) onto the DSBs. This is also true in the case of ATR-deleted mammalian cells *(291)*. Now the question arises whether all these proteins in replication or DNA damage sites are recruited to the DNA or loaded onto the DNA–protein complexes. DNA polymerase α (primase) initiates replication by synthesizing an RNA primer, which is subsequently elongated by DNA polymerase α. RFC associates with DNA during replication. In yeast, checkpoint-defective alleles of primase have been identified *(292)*. In vitro reconstitution of the checkpoint in *Xenopus* extracts also requires RNA primer *(293,294)*. Thus, it will be of interest to discover whether primase promotes the loading of ATM or ATR or the 9-1-1 complexes at the damage site, and whether primase has any role in loading these proteins onto the replication machinery.

9.4. DNA Repair As a Complex Process Coupled With Checkpoint Function

Before DNA replication in normal cells, DNA lesions are removed either by nucleotide-excision or base-excision repair (NER or BER) pathways. A third kind of repair also exists, which corrects bases that are mispaired owing to faulty DNA replication; this is known as mismatch repair (MMR) *(295)*. If the DNA is not repaired by the above pathways, replication forks accumulate at the site of DNA damage and activate the postreplication repair pathways. Two modes of postreplication repair exist in cellular systems. DNA polymerases that involve the error-prone mode of repair read through the sites of DNA lesion, whereas the error-free mode of DNA repair proceeds through a template-switching event involving the undamaged sister chromatid. Once DNA damage is recognized, a checkpoint has to be triggered, followed by DNA repair *(295–298)*. In BER, a DNA glycosylase binds selectively to an altered nucleotide and cleaves the *N*-glycosylic bond between the base and the deoxyribose sugar. Other enzymes, such as AP lyase, AP endonuclease, and DNA polymerase, load onto the free ribose overhang and repair the nicked site *(297,298)*. NER acts on bulky DNA lesions such as DNA adducts, formed by benzo (a) pyrene, or pyrimidine dimers, formed by UV. This abnormality is found in Xeroderma pigmentosum and Cockayne's syndrome patients *(299)*. Bacteria use the UvrABC complex, whereas eukaryotes have evolved the XPC–HR23B protein complex, which is homologous to the yeast Rad4–Rad23 complex. Along with XPC–HR23B, other proteins, including XPA, XPE, the single-stranded DNA binding factor, the replication protein A (RPA), and the basal transcription factor TFIIA (contains the helicases XPB and XPD), bind to DNA for recognition and verification of DNA lesions and for recruiting other NERs. NERs occur in two ways: either on the silent or nontranscribed strand of the active gene (global genomic repair), or on the transcribed strand of the gene (transcription coupled repair), where RNA polymerase elongation is blocked by DNA damage *(300,301)*. Similarly, MMR pathways use the MSH 2, 3, and 6 proteins, which recognize mispaired DNA *(302,303)*. MSH2–MSH6 recognizes the mismatched bases or small insertions or deletion loops, whereas MSH2–MSH3 detects only larger loops. In *E. coli*, the MutS homodimer binds to the DNA mismatch or loop, followed by MutL loading which, in the presence of ATP, makes an incision on the daughter strand at a d(GATC) site by MutH. After nick formation, DNA helicase II (UvrD/MutU) displaces the strand, which is subsequently degraded by one of the four exonucleases: RecJ, ExoVII, ExoI, or ExoX *(304)*. UV and alkylation damage can be repaired by direct reversal by O^6-alkyguanine alkyl transferase *(305)*. Dioxygenases ABH1 and ABH3 catalyze the oxidation and release of a methyl group from 1-methyladenine and 3-methylcytosine *(306)*. Methyl transferase can also catalyze the methyl group from O^4methylthymine *(307)*. However, in yeast, plants, and bacteria, UV damage can be repaired by the enzyme photolyase through photoreactivation *(308)*. RNAPs act as recognition factors for TCR (transcription coupled repair) in transcription arrest. Mammalian RNAPs I and III do not elicit TCR in mammals, but RNAP II does *(309,310)*. These arrested RNAPs in human cells produce signals for apoptosis *(295,311)*. Thus, the RNAP II signals DNA repair and also prevents cell death. Similarly, the ssDNA-binding protein, RPA, is required for the assembly of DNA-polymerase-α with primase at replication origins for initiation of replication and synthesis of nascent DNA. It also binds to other types of DNA lesions *(295,312)*. In NER, RPA interacts through XPA, XPG, and the XPF–ERCC complex *(313–315)*. RPA along with XPA fully opens the DNA double helix and sites of DNA damage by TFIIH. RPA also likely positions the repair endonucleases through the interaction with

XPG on its 3' side and XPF–ERCC on its 5'-facing end. The role of RPA is complex, and many questions remain to be answered. If RPA is the first to bind to the DNA damage, how does it normally function in the absence of damage? How does RPA interact or crosstalk with several repair proteins? Does DNA-damage-dependent phosphorylation of RPA alter normal cellular growth to a repair function? Is ATR kinase involved in this process to maintain the checkpoint function as well as the repair of damaged DNA? It is possible that the level of DNA damage in the cell might be an important factor to decide which complex will be loaded to the chromatin? At low levels of damage, before the checkpoint proteins act, the repair proteins may repair the damage. However, if the damage is high, then checkpoint proteins sense the damage and pass signals to arrest the cells.

The transcription factor BRCA1 not only acts as a co-activator of p53, but also acts in tandem with the survival and repair pathway, but not with the apoptosis pathway *(316)*. BRCA1 co-localizes with macroH2A1, H3mK9 (histone methylated at Lys9) at the inactive X *(317)*, and H2AX (γ-H2AX) phosphorylated at Ser139, after DNA damage *(318)*. H2AX gets phosphorylated after DNA damage, showing discrete foci within 10 min of DNA damage. However, BRCA1 loaded to this complex after 30 min followed by RAD50/RAD51 also co-localizes with DNA damage-induced foci *(317–318)*. Thus, H2AX is not only upstream of BRCA1 but also may be a DNA damage sensor *(316)*. H2AX-null cells are hypersensitive to IR and have increased spontaneous chromosome aberrations *(319,320)*. Similarly, BRCA1-deficient cells have defects in DNA damage-repair pathways and have defects in transcription-coupled repair, homologous recombination, nonhomologous end-joining, and microhomology end-joining *(321–323)*. The binding of BRCA1 with the repair genes suggests that either it indirectly regulates the pathways or may act through transcription or ubiquitination mechanisms.

9.5. DNA Damage-Dependent G1 Checkpoint

G1 phase is a period when cells carry out processes necessary to enter the next stage for the completion of DNA synthesis and, ultimately, mitotic exit. This critical point, where the cell can either stop or go to the next phase, is called the restriction point between mid to late G1 phase *(324)*. However, even if cells pass the restriction point, a stress signal alarms the cells not to cross the G1–S transition. There are many transcription factors that can regulate genes involved in this response. Phosphorylation of Rb by cyclin D–Cdk4/6 kinase is one of the critical factors in the G1/S transition *(112,324)*. Phosphorylated Rb is released from the E2F family of transcription factors, which heterodimerize with the DP proteins and initiate S phase through activation of gene expression. These heterodimeric transcription factors lead to the expression of dihydrofolate reductase, thymidine kinase, thymidylate synthase, and DNA polymerase alpha *(69)*. In addition, cyclin E–Cdk2 and cyclin A–Cdk2 are activated to allow progress through the transition point. However, if there is DNA damage before the cells transit through the G1/S checkpoint, transcription factor p53 not only translocates to the nucleus but also activates the downstream target Cdk inhibitor p21, which inactivates cyclin E–Cdk2 kinase activity and causes cell cycle arrest at the G1/S transition *(20,59,60,325,326)*. Similarly, E2F and Myc activate cyclin E, and levels of cyclin E are detectable in late G1 *(231)*. Both Cdk2 and RB are also targeted by the DNA damage checkpoint *(327–329)*. Thus, the position and its application in the Rb and Myc convergence makes cyclin E–Cdk2 a DNA damage checkpoint target *(231)*. However, inactivity of cyclin E–Cdk2 also occurs at late G1 in p53- or p21-null cells, suggesting that there are other ways in which the G1 cell cycle proceeds. The initial checkpoint is rapid, transient, and p53 independent, after which p53-p21 sustains and prolongs G1 arrest.

9.6. p53-Independent G1 Checkpoint

In the normal course of cell cycle progression, the phosphatase Cdc25A dephosphorylates inhibitory residues on Cdk2 and allows cells to proceed to S phase *(231)*. However, in mammalian cells exposed to UV or IR, the levels of Cdc25A decrease by ubiquitination and rapid protein turnover by the proteasomes *(327–329)*. Thus, inactivation of Cdc25A mediates a checkpoint pathway where Cdk2 inhibitory tyrosine 15 persists and blocks the G1/S transition. UV or IR exposure results in Cdc25A phosphorylation at serine 123, either by Chk1 or Chk2, and this is sensitive to caffeine, an inhibitor of ATM/ATR *(329,330)*. By blocking the degradation of Cdc25A, the rate of DNA damage increases and cell survival decreases *(327)*. The endpoint of this pathway is the inhibition of Cdk2-dependent loading of Cdc45 to the DNA prereplication complexes. Thus, the ATM/ATR-Chk2/Chk1-Cdc25A-Cdk2 pathway is independent of p53, and this occurs by a cascade of protein–protein interactions, phosphorylation, ubiquitination, and proteolysis of the key target, Cdc25A. IR also results in degradation of cyclin D1, another G1 regulator, but not the D2 and D3 cyclins. Simultaneously, the assembly factor p21 translocates from the cyclin D–Cdk4/6 complex to the cyclin E–Cdk2 complex to inhibit G1–S progression. This is an ATM-independent DNA damage G1 checkpoint. However, IR also degrades Cdc25A through ubiquitination, and this process is conserved from *Xenopus* to mammals *(327–329)*.

9.7. Posttranslational Modification of p53 and G1 Arrest

DNA damage causes activation of p53, and this causes repression or activation of more than 150 genes *(20,331–333)*. The action of p53 is increased many fold after its modification by phosphorylation at different serine sites, mainly at Ser 6, 9, 15, 20, 33, 37, 46, and Thr 18 and Thr 81 at the N-terminal end. Similarly, in the C-terminal regulatory domain, Ser 315 and 392 are phosphorylated, Lys 320, 373, and 382 are acetylated, and Lys 386 is sumoylated in response to DNA damage *(334)*. In contrast, Thr 55 and Ser 376 and 378 are constitutively phosphorylated in normal cells *(335)*. Thr 55 dephosphorylation occurs after DNA damage *(335)*. ATM and Chk2 activate p53 in response to IR, while ATR and Chk1 appear to be required for the response to UV damage *(268,336–338)*. The DNA damage-dependent G1 arrest is mainly p53 dependent. ATM phosphorylates p53 at serine 15 and enhances the transcriptional activity of p53, which causes p21 transcriptional activation *(336,337)*. Similarly, ATM targets Chk2, which in turn phosphorylates p53 at Ser 20 *(337)*. The phosphorylation of p53 interferes with the Mdm2 interaction that leads to p53 stabilization. Similarly, ATM also phosphorylates Mdm2 on Ser 395 *(339)*. This interferes with the nuclear export of p53–Mdm2 and hence p53 degradation through ubiquitination. Although ATM phosphorylates p53 on Ser 9 and Ser 46 and dephosphorylates it on Ser 376, the functional significance of this is still unknown *(340)*.

9.8. DNA Damage and Intra-S-Phase Checkpoint

ATM phosphorylates the tumor suppressor protein Brca1 on several sites *(341–343)*; this process is also involved in the S phase and G2/M checkpoint *(345)*. The Ser 1387 of Brca1 acts as a regulator of an intra-S phase checkpoint *(346)*. Chk2 also phosphorylates Brca1 *(347)*. ATM regulates Brca1 function through phosphorylation of two residues of CtIP, an inhibitor of Brca1 *(348)*. Besides Brca1, ATM also phosphorylates structural maintenance of chromosomes-1 (SMC1) on two serine residues, and blocking these phosphorylations abrogates the intra-S phase checkpoint **(Fig. 8)** *(349,350)*. Fanconi's anemia syndrome protein (FANCD2), an effector of ATM in the intra-S phase checkpoint, is phosphorylated on Ser 222 by ATM and undergoes Brca1-mediated mono-ubiquitination *(351)*. There is also evidence that to maintain the replication checkpoint, the phosphorylation of Cdc25 phosphatase by Cds1or Chk1 is required *(352)*. The role of Chk1 in stabilizing Cdc25A, which activates cyclin E–Cdk2 activity at multiple cell cycle checkpoints including the S or replication checkpoint, has been revealed in vertebrate cells *(233)*. Overexpression of *cdc25A* abrogates checkpoint-induced S phase arrest *(353)*. Cdc25A is degraded in response to UV light or drugs that block DNA replication *(327)*. The block in DNA replication activates ATR-Chk1 activity, and the latter probably phosphorylates Cdc25A at Ser 123, resulting in rapid degradation of Cdc25A and S phase arrest *(329)*. A similar Ser 123 phosphorylation by IR-induced DNA damage and subsequent degradation of Cdc25A has been reported through ATM-Cds1, but is not likely by Chk1 *(273)*. However, Chk1-deficient cells fail to show rapid degradation of Cdc25A, suggesting that both ATM-Cds1 and ATR-Chk1 may mediate phosphorylation of Cdc25A, resulting in the degradation of the protein and the establishment of an S phase checkpoint *(273)*.

9.9. Serine/Threonine Kinases and DNA Damage G2/M Checkpoint

In mammalian cells, G2 arrest is mainly regulated by the cyclin B/Cdc2 inhibitory phosphorylations, and this can be overcome by the activation of the phosphatases Cdc25A, B, and C. Cdc25A binds and activates the cyclin B–Cdc2 kinase, and its absence delays entry into mitosis *(1–3,354)*. Overexpression of Cdc25A abrogates G2 arrest, while DNA damage results in degradation of Cdc25A, and Chk1 is required for G2 arrest and degradation *(273,354–356)*. Interphase cells have the Ser-216-phosphorylated form of Cdc25. The mitotic form of Cdc25 lacks the Ser 216 phosphorylation, and this is the active form *(354)*. Following DNA damage, Chk1 or Chk2 phosphorylates Cdc25 at Ser 216, which leads to binding of 14-3-3 proteins and sequestration in the cytoplasm *(234,354–357)*. This causes Cdk inactivation and G2/M arrest. Cdc25C phosphorylation by Chk2 acts at the G2/M transition *(254,255)*. Chk1 is the preferred ATR target in the G2/M pathway, and ATR also prevents premature chromatin condensation *(234,354,355)*. The evidence is that a serine 216 to alanine mutant does not completely rescue the G2/M arrest *(355)*. In addition, Cdc25C localization is not sufficient or necessary for checkpoint function *(356,357)*. A role of Cds1 in G2/M arrest was proposed on the basis of fission yeast in which genetic and biochemical analyses demonstrated the action of Cdc25 in checkpoint regulation *(358,359)*. Further results from different groups argue that Cds1/Chk1 phosphorylates more residues by which Cdc25 loses phosphatase activity, and the activity is suppressed until the checkpoint signals vanish following DNA damage *(355)*. However, a Chk2 role in Cdc25 inactivation has been ruled out partly because Cds1-knockout mice arrest cells in G2 for 12 h following γ irradiation *(259)*. But at the same time, it might be acting in the maintenance of the arrest, as Chk2–/– mice do not maintain well an initial arrest after irradiation *(259)*. Similarly, in somatic cells, p53 is required to sustain a long-term G2 arrest after IR *(259)*. Phosphorylation of Brca1 by ATM on Ser 1432 is one of the targets at the G2/M checkpoint, suggesting different sites of Brca1 play a different role in different checkpoints *(360)*. Brca1-deficient mice fail to arrest cells in G2, fail in transcription-coupled repair, and have impaired homologous recombination repair pathways following IR, suggesting a major role in G2 checkpoint and repair pathways *(361)*. Polo-like kinases play multiple roles in DNA damage checkpoints in G2 arrest, mitosis, and in mitotic exit *(90)*. Although Plk1 does not directly control a G2 checkpoint, Cdc5, the homolog of Plk1, can prevent anaphase entry to mitotic exits in response to DNA damage in budding yeast *(362,363)*. Plk1 activates Cdc25C, as in *Xenopus* depletion of Plk1 causes a block in Cdc25C activation, and cell cycle arrest. On the other hand, overexpression of a mutant form of Plk1 can overcome G2 arrest caused by DNA damage, suggesting a role for Plk1 in the DNA damage checkpoint *(365)*.

10. Checkpoint Defects and Cancer

Genetic instability is one of the hallmarks of cancer, and its links to mutations in a number of checkpoint genes, aberrations in DNA repair machinery, and the cell cycle checkpoint pathways is well documented *(1–10)* However, the defects in checkpoints that result in predisposition to and diagnosis of cancer will be discussed elsewhere. Here, we focus on the significance of the defects with respect to cell cycle checkpoints and cancer. Except for ATR and Chk1, whose knockout causes embryonic lethality in mice, all the major G1/S checkpoint transducers and effectors can act as tumor suppressors or proto-oncogenes, depending on whether they promote or inhibit cell cycle progression. Genes that are mutated in human tumors are listed in **Table 2** *(366–375)*.

A number of genes, including p53, Rb, Ras, and so on, cause abnormal growth when mutated, either because of loss of tumor-suppressive or gain of growth-promoting activities. Absence of p53, the most commonly mutated gene in human cancer, has a major effect on cell cycle checkpoint regulators, as it transactivates a number of genes, including the growth-inhibitory gene p21 and a number of apoptotic genes, particularly after DNA damage-induced G1 block. In a similar manner, G1 restriction-point disruption in some tumors results in an unlimited growth through overexpression of certain checkpoint genes, such as cyclin D in parathyroid adenomas or cyclin E in breast cancer. Cyclin D mutation is also common in some sporadic cancer cases, consistence with its pivotal role in the G1 restriction point. A new inhibitory protein of Cdk2, called Cables, has been reported to be inactivated in 50–60% of primary colon and head and neck tumors *(369)*. Further, hereditary mutations that predispose to cancer include p53, BRCA1, p16, Rb, Mre11, Nbs1, ATM, and Chk2 *(7,14,20,21,24,72,149,230–233,267,269,272,295,316,323,324, 327,331,345,350,361,366)*. Loss of p16INK4A in different tumors, and also p15INK4B and p14ARF, a positive regulator of p53, eliminates the action of cyclin-kinase inhibitors at G1/S progression *(7,367)*. Lower expression, degradation, and mislocalization of the p27 cyclin-kinase inhibitor has been shown to be important in G1/S regulation *(7,368)*. Deregulation of Rb function by HPV E7, SV40 T antigen, and adenovirus E1A, observed in different tumor samples, suggests the importance of Rb in uncontrolled cell division and tumor formation *(24,367)*. Chk2 mutations occur in Li–Fraumeni syndrome, while inherited p53 mutations were not observed in these same families *(369)*. The genomic instability syndromes, including xeroderma pigmentosum, Cockayne's syndrome, trichothiodystrophy, Bloom's syndrome, Werner's syn-

Table 2
Defects in Some of the G1/S/G2-M Checkpoint Genes in Different Tumors

Gene/protein	Molecular aberrations	Tumor type(s)
p53	M, D, VI	all cancers
Cyclin D1	A, T, HE	many cancers
Cyclin E	A, HE	breast and ovarian cancer
Rb	VI, D, T, F, A	many cancers
p16	D, M, PS	many cancers
Cdc25A	HE	breast cancers
BRCA1	M, D, F, T	breast, ovarian cancer
ATM	D, M, T, LE	breast cancer, lymphoma
Chk1	F	colon, endometrial cancer
Chk2	M, T, D, LE	breast, colon, lung, testis, urinary bladder carcinoma
Mre11	M, F, T	breast, lymphoid tumors
Nbs1	T	unknown
hBub1	D, T	colon, lung cancer
Chfr	Methylation	Colon, non-small-cell lung cancer

Abbreviations: D = deletion; M = missense mutation; F = frame-shift mutation; T = transloca-tion; T = truncation; A = amplification; PS = promoter silencing; LE = lower expression; HE = higher expression; VI = virus mediated inactivation.

drome, Rothmund–Thompson syndrome, and Fanconi's anemia, affect DNA damage-response pathways, causing abnormal genomic repair and cell divison, either directly or indirectly. Some of these have a predisposition to cancer fol-lowing ionizing/UV radiation or certain chemicals. The HTLV-1 virus for faster multiplication of the virus targeted Mad1, the mitotic checkpoint gene *(370)*. Similarly, securin (the pituitary tumor-transforming gene, PTTG) chro-mosome segregation protein has transformation ability, besides being overexpressed in cancer cell lines *(371)*. Further, people with Mad2 haplo-insufficiency have been reported to have checkpoint defects and to be suscep-tible to lung cancer in later life. Bub1 and BubR1 mutations also cooperate with the BRCA2 deficiency in the pathogenesis of breast cancer. In addition *(372–374)*, Bub1 mutants are responsible for a chromosome instability pheno-type in certain colorectal and lung tumors *(375)*. The prometaphase checkpoint gene Chfr also seems to be hypermethylated in many cancers, including colon, brain, bone, and non-small-cell lung carcinoma, and treatment with 5-aza-2'-deoxycytidine results in partial restoration of a prophase checkpoint, suggest-ing the importance of this protein in mitotic arrest *(376)*.

3. Morgan, D. O. (1999) Regulation of APC and the exit from mitosis. *Nat. Cell. Biol.* **2,** E47–53

4. Pines, J. (1999) Four-dimensional control of the cell cycle. *Nat. Cell. Biol.* **1,** E73–79.

5. Hartwell, L. H. and Weinert, T. A. (1989) Checkpoints: controls that ensure the order of cell cycle events. *Science* **246,** 629–634.

6. Weinert, T. A. and Hartwell, L. H. (1988) The RAD9 gene controls the cell cycle response to DNA damage in *Saccharomyces cerevisiae. Science* **246,** 317–322.

7. McDonald III, E. R. and El-Deiry, W. S. (2001) Checkpoint genes in cancer. *Ann. Med.* **33,** 113–122.

8. Nasmyth, K. (1996) Viewpoint: putting the cell cycle in order. *Science* **274,** 1643–1645.

9. Pardee, A. B. (1989) G1 events and regulation of cell proliferation. *Science* **246,** 603–608.

10. King, R. W., Jackson, P.A., and Kirschner, M. W. (1994) Mitosis in transition. *Cell* **79,** 563–571.

11. King, R. W., Deshaies, R. J., Peters, J. M., and Kirshner, M. W. (1996) How proteolysis drives the cell cycle. *Science* **274,** 1652–1659.

12. Shapiro, J. A. and Harper, J. W. (1999) Anticancer drug targets: cell cycle and checkpoint control. *J. Clin. Invest.* **104,** 1645–1653.

13. Hahn, W. C., Counter, C. M., Lundberg, A. S., Beijersbergen, R. L., Brooks, M. W., and Weinberg, R. A. (1999) Creation of human tumor cells with defined genetic elements. *Nature* **400,** 464–468.

14. Vogelstein, B. and Kinzler, K. W. (1993) The multistep nature of cancer. *Trends in Genet.* **9,** 138–141.

15. Hayflick, L. and Moorhead, P. S. (1961) The serial cultivation of human diploid cell strains. *Exp. Cell Res.* **25,** 585–621.

16. Lingner, J., Hughes, T. R., Shevchenko, A., Mann, M., Lundblad, V., and Cech, T. R. (1997) Reverse transcriptase motifs in the catalytic subunit of telomerase. *Science* **276,** 561–567.

17. Bodnar, A. G., Ouellette, M., Frolkis, M., et al. (1998) Extension of life-span by introduction of telomerase into normal human cells. *Science* **279,** 349–352.

18. Hanahan, D. and Weinberg, R. A. (2000) The hallmarks of cancer. *Cell* **100,** 57–70.

19. Pearson, M., Carbone, R., Sebastiani, C., et al. (2000) PML regulates p53 acetylation and premature senescence induced by oncogenic Ras. *Nature* **406,** 207–210.

20. El-Deiry, W. S. (1998) Regulation of p53 downstream genes. *Semin. Cancer Biol.* **8,** 345–357.

21. Ozoren, N. and El-Deiry, W. S. (2000) Introduction to cancer genes and growth control. In: *DNA Alterations in Cancer Genetic and Epigenetic Changes* (Ehrlich, M., ed.), Eaton Publishing, Natick, MA: pp. 3–43.

22. Hunter, T. (1997) Oncoprotein networks. *Cell* **88,** 333–346.

23. Elledge, S. and Spottswood, M. (1991) A new human p34 protein kinase, CDK2, identified by complementation of a *cdc28* mutation in *Saccharomyces cerevisiae,* is a homolog of *Xenopus* Eg1. *EMBO J.* **10,** 2653–2659.

24. McDonald, E. R. 3rd and El-Deiry, W. S. (2000) Cell cycle control as a basis for cancer drug development (Review). *Int. J. Onco.* **16,** 871–886.

25. Oehlen, L. J., Jeoung, D. I., and Cross, F. R. (1998) Cyclin-specific START events and the G1-phase specificity of arrest by mating factor in budding yeast. *Mol. Gen. Genet.* **258,** 183–189.

26. Schwob, E. and Nasmyth, K. (1993) CLB5 and CLB6, a new pair of B cyclins involved in DNA replication in *Saccharomyces cerevisiae. Genes Dev.* **7,** 1160–1175.

27. Fisher, D. L. and Nurse, P. (1996) A single fission yeast mitotic cyclin B p34cdc2 kinase promotes both S-phase and mitosis in the absence of G1 cyclins. *EMBO J.* **15,** 850–860.

28. Levine, K., Huang, K., and Cross, F. R. (1996) *Saccharomyces cerevisiae* G1 cyclins differ in their intrinsic functional specificities. *Mol. Cell. Biol.* **271,** 25240–25246.

29. Tetsu, O. and McCormick, F. (2003) Proliferation of cancer cells despite Cdk2 inhibition. *Cancer Cell* **3,** 233–245.

30. Baldin, V., Lukas, J., Marcote, M. J., Pgano, M., and Draetta, G. (1993) Cyclin D1 is a nuclear protein required for cell cycle progression in G1. *Genes Dev.* **7,** 812–821.

31. Lukas, J., Bartkova, J., Rhode, M., Strauss, M., and Bartek, J. (1995) Cyclin D1 is dispensable for G1 control in retinoblastoma gene-deficient cells, independently of Cdk4 activity. *Mol. Cell. Biol.* **15,** 2600–2611.

32. Ohtsubo, M., Theodoras, A. M., Schumacher, J., Roberts, J. M., and Pagano, M. (1995) Human cyclin E, a nuclear protein essential for the G1-to-S phase transition. *Mol. Cell. Biol.* **15,** 2612–2624.

33. Geng, Y., Whoriskey, W., Park, M., et al. (1999) Rescue of cyclin D1 deficiency by knockin cyclin E. *Cell* **97,** 767–777.

34. Girard, F., Strausfeld, U., Fernandez, A., and Lamb, N. J. C. (1992) Cylcin A is required for the onset of DNA replication in mammalian fibroblast. *Cell* **67,** 1169–1179.

35. Pagano, M., Pepperkok, F., Verde, F., Ansorge, W., and Draetta, G. (1992) Cyclin A is required at two points in the human cell cycle. *EMBO J.* **11,** 961–971.

36. Geng, Y., Yu, Q., Sicinska, E., et al. (2003) Cyclin E ablation in the mouse. *Cell* **114,** 431–443.

36a. Roberts, J. M. and Sherr, C. J. (2003) Bared essentials of CDK2 and cyclin E. *Nat. Genet.* **35,** 9–10.

37. Murphy, M., Stinnakre, M.-G., Senamaud-Beaufort, C., et al. (1997) Delayed early embryonic lethality following disruption of the murine cyclin A2 gene. *Nat. Genet.* **15,** 83–86.

38. Brandeis, M., Rosewell, I., Carrington, M., et al. (1998) Cyclin B2–null mice develop normally and are fertile whereas cyclin B1–null mice die in utero. *Proc. Natl. Acad. Sci. USA* **95,** 4344–4349.

39. Kaffman, A., Herskowitz, I., Tjian, R., and O'Shea, E. K. (1994) Phosphorylation of the transcription factor PHO4 by a cyclin–CDK complex, PHO80–PHO85. *Science* **263,** 1153–1156.

73. Kellogg, D. R., Mortiz, M., and Alberts, B. M. (1994) The centrosome and cellular organization. *Annu. Rev. Biochem.* **63,** 639–674

74. Okuda, G., Horn, H. F., Tarapore, P., et al. (2000) Nucleophosmin/B23 is a target of Cdk2/cylin E in centrosome duplication. *Cell* **103,** 127–140.

75. Fisk, H. A. and Winey, M. (2001) The mouse mps1p-like kinase regulates centrosome duplication. *Cell* **106,** 95–104.

76. Stucke, V. M., Sillje, H. H. W., Arnaud, L., and Nigg, E. A. (2002) Human Mps1 kinase is required for the spindle assembly checkpoint but not for centrosome duplication. *EMBO J.* **21,** 1723–1732.

77. Hinchcliffe, E. H., Miller, F. J., Cham, M., Khodjakov, A., and Sluder, G. (2001) Requirement of a centrosomal activity for cell cycle progression through G1 to S phase. *Science* **291,** 1547–1550.

78. Piel, M., Nordberg, J., Euteneuer, U., and Bornens, M. (2001) Centrosome-dependent exit of cytokinesis in animal cells. *Science* **291,** 1550–1553.

79. Doxsey, S. (2001) Re-evaluating centrosome function. *Nature Rev.* **2,** 688–698.

80. Lane, H. A. and Nigg, E. A. (1996) Antibody microinjection reveals an essential role for human polo-like kinase (Plk1) in the functional maturation of mitotic centrosomes. *J. Cell. Biol.* **135,** 1701–1713.

81. do Carno-Avides, M. and Glover, D. M. (1999) Abnormal spindle protein, Asp, and the integrity of mitotic centrosomal microtubule organizing centers. *Science* **283,** 1733–1735.

82. Fry, A. M., Meraldi, P., and Nigg, E. A. (1998) A centrosomal function for the human Nek2 protein kinase, a member of the NIMA family of cell cycle regulators. *EMBO J.* **17,** 470–481.

83. Helps, N. R., Luo, X., Barker, H. M., and Cohen, P. T. (2000) NIMA-related kinase 2 (Nek2), a cell-cycle-regulated protein kinase localized to centrosomes, is complexed to protein phosphatase 1. *Biochem. J.* **349,** 509–518.

84. Blangy, A., Lane, H. A., d'Herin, P., Harper, M., Kress, M., and Nigg, E. A. (1995) Phosphorylation by p34cdc2 regulates spindle association of human Eg5, a kinesin-related motor essential for bipolar spindle formation in vivo. *Cell* **83,** 1159–1169.

85. Giet, R., Uzbekov, R., Cubizolles, F., Le Guellec, K., and Prigent, C. (1999) The *Xenopus laevis* aurora-related protein kinase pEg2 associates with and phosphorylates the kinesin-related protein XIEg5. *JBC* **272,** 19418–19424.

86. Meraldi, P. and Nigg, E. A. (2002) The centrosome cycle. *FEBS Lett.* **521,** 9–13.

87. Schumacher, J. M., Ashcroft, N., Donovan, P. J., and Golden, A. (1998) A highly conserved centrosomal kinase, AIR-1, is required for accurate cell cycle progression and segregation of developmental factors in *Caenorhabditis elegans* embryos. *Development* **125,** 4391–4402.

88. Nigg, E. A. (1995) Cyclin-dependent protein kinases: key regulators of the eukaryotic cell cycle. *Bioessays* **17,** 471–480.

89. Meraldi, P. and Nigg, E. A. (2002) The centrosome cycle, *FEBS Lett.* **521,** 9–13.

90. Nigg, E. A. (2001) Mitotic kinases as regulators of cell division and its checkpoints. *Nat. Rev. Mol. Cell. Biol.* **2,** 21–32.

91. Kramer, A., Neben, K., and Ho A. D. (2002) Centrosome replication, genomic instability and cancer. *Leukemia* **16,** 767–775.

92. Tarapore, P., Horn, H. F., Tokuyama, Y., and Fukasawa, K. (2001) Direct regulation of the centrosome duplication cycle by the p53–p21 Waf1/cip1 pathway. *Oncogene* **20,** 3173–3184.

93. Zhou, H., Kuang, J., Zhong, L., et al. (1998) Tumour amplified kinase STK15/BTAK induces centrosome amplification, aneuploidy and transformation. *Nat. Genet.* **20,** 189–193.

94. Koshland, D. and Strunnikov, A. (1996) Mitotic chromosome condensation. *Annu. Rev. Cell Dev. Biol.* **12,** 305–333.

95. Cheung, P., Alis, D. C., and Sassone-Cors, P. (2000) Signaling to chromatin through histone modifications. *Cell* **103,** 263–271.

96. Goto, H., Tomono, Y., Ajiro, K., et al. (1999) Identification of a novel phosphorylation site on histone H3 coupled with mitotic chromosome condensation. *JBC* **274,** 25543–25549.

97. Kimura, K., Hirano, M., Kobayashi, R., and Hirano, T. (1998) Phosphorylation and activation of 13S condensin by Cdc2 in vitro. *Science* **282,** 487–490.

98. Evans, T., Rosenthal, E. T., Youngbloom, J., Distel, D., and Hunt, T. (1983) Cyclin: a protein specified by maternal mRNA in sea urchin eggs that is destroyed at each cleavage division. *Cell* **33,** 389–396.

99. Thomas, G. (2000) An encore for ribosome biogenesis in the control of cell proliferation. *Nat. Cell Biol.* **2,** E71–E72.

100. Schmelzle, T. and Hall, M. N. (2000) TOR, a central controller of cell growth. *Cell* **103,** 253–262.

101. Rhode, J., Heitman, J., and Cardenas, M. E. (2001) The TOR kinases link nutrient sensing to cell growth. *JBC* **276,** 9583–9586.

102. Fukunaga, R. and Hunter, T. (1997) MNK1, a new MAP kinase activated protein kinase, isolated by a novel expression screening method for identifying protein kinase substrates. *EMBO J.* **16,** 1921–1933.

103. Waskiewicz, A. J., Flynn, A., Proud, C. G., and Cooper, J. A. (1997) Mitogen-activated protein kinases activate the serine/threonine kinases Mnk1 and Mnk2. *EMBO J.* **16,** 1909–1920.

104. Malumbres, M. and Pellicer, A. (1998) Ras pathways to cell cycle control and cell transformation. *Front. Biosci.* **3,** D887–D912.

105. Ganoth, D., Bomstein, G., Ko, T. K., Larsen, B., Tyers, M., and Pagano, M. (2001) The cell-cycle regulatory protein Cks1 is required for SCF (Skp2)-mediated ubiquitinylation of p27. *Nat. Cell Biol.* **3,** 321–324.

106. Webley, K., Bond, J. A., Jones, C. J., et al. (2000) Posttranslational modifications of p53 in replicative senescence overlapping but distinct from those induced by DNA damage. *Mol. Cell. Biol.* **20,** 2830–2838.

107. Baluchamy, S., Rjabi, H., Thimmapaya, R., Navaraj, A., and Thimmapaya, B. (2003) Repression of c-Myc and inhibition of G1 exit in cells conditionally overexpressing p300 that is not dependent on its histone acetyltransferase activity. *Proc. Nat. Acad. Sci. USA* **100,** 9524–9529.

108. Lavita, P. and Jansen-Durr, P. (1999) E2F target genes and cell-cycle checkpoint control. *Bioessays* **21,** 221–230.
109. Lundberg, A. S. and Weinberg, R. A. (1998) Functional inactivation of the retinoblastoma protein requires sequential modification by at least two distinct cyclin–CDK complexes. *Mol. Cell. Biol.* **18,** 753–761.
110. Harbour, J. W., Luo, R. X., Dei Santi, A., Postigo, A. A., and Dean, D. C. (1999) Cdk phosphorylation triggers sequential intramolecular interactions that progressively block Rb functions as cells move through G1. *Cell* **98,** 859–869.
111. Ezhevsky, S. A., Ho, A., Becker-Hapak, M., Davis, P. K., and Dowdy, S. F. (2001) Differential regulation of retinoblastoma tumor suppressor protein by G1 cyclin-dependent kinase complexes in vivo. *Mol. Cell. Biol.* **21,** 4773–4784.
112. Sherr, C. J. and Roberts, J. M. (1999) Cdk inhibitors: positive and negative regulators of G1-phase progression. *Genes and Dev.* **13,** 1501–1512.
113. Chan, H. M., Kristic-Demonacos, M., Smith, L., Demonacos, C., and La Thangue, N. B. (2001) Acetylation control of the retinoblastoma tumour-suppressor protein. *Nat. Cell Bio.* **3,** 667–674.
114. Strohmaier, H., Spruck, C. H., Kaiser, P., Won, K. A., Sangfelt, O., and Reed S. I. (2001) Human F-box protein hCdc4 targets cyclin E for proteolysis and is mutated in a breast cancer cell line. *Nature* **413,** 316–322.
115. Koepp, D. M., Schaefer, L. K., Ye, X., Keyomarsi, K., Chu, C., and Harper, J. W. (2001) Phosphorylation-dependent ubiquitination of cyclin E by the SCF^Fbw7 ubiquitin ligase. *Science* **294,** 173–177.
116. Welcker, M., Singer, J., Loeb, K. R., et al. (2003) Multisite phosphorylation by Cdk2 and GSK3 controls cyclin E degradation. *Mol. Cell* **12,** 381–392.
117. Krek, W., Ewen, M. E., Shirodkar, S., Arany, Z., Kaelin, W. G., and Livingston, D. M. (1994) Negative regulation of the growth-promoting transcription factor E2F-1 by a stably bound cyclin A–dependent protein kinase. *Cell* **78,** 161–172.
118. Krek, W., Xu, G., and Livingston, D. M. (1995) Cyclin A kinase regulation of E2F-1 DNA binding function underlies suppression of an S phase checkpoint. *Cell* **83,** 1149–1158.
119. Dynlacht, B. D., Flores, O., Lees, J. A., and Harlow, E. (1994) Differential regulation of E2F transactivation by cyclin/cdk2 complexes. *Genes Dev.* **8,** 1772–1786.
120. Nguyen, V. Q., Co, C., and Li, J. J. (2001) Cyclin-dependent kinases prevent DNA re-replication through multiple mechanisms. *Nature* **411,** 1068–1073.
121. Yanow, S. K., Lygerou, Z., and Nurse, P. (2001) Expression of Cdc18/Cdc6 and Cdt1 during G2 phase induces initiation of DNA replication. *EMBO J.* **20,** 4648–4656.
122. Stillman, B. (1996) Cell cycle control of DNA replication. *Science* **274,** 1659–1664.
123. Bell, S. P. and Dutta, A. (2002) DNA replication in eukaryotic cells. *Ann. Rev. Biochem.* **71,** 333–374.
124. Delmolino, L. M., Saha, P., and Dutta, A. (2001) Multiple mechanisms regulate subcellular localization of human CDC6. *JBC* **276,** 26947–26954.
125. Mendez, J. and Stillman, B. (2000) Chromatin association of human origin recognition complex, cdc6, and minichromosome maintenance proteins during the cell cycle: assembly of prereplication complexes in late mitosis. *Mol. Cell. Biol.* **20,** 8602–8612.

126. Pelizon, C., Madine, M. A., Romanowski, P., and Lskey, R. A., (2000) Unphosphorylatable mutants of Cdc6 disrupt its nuclear export but still support DNA replication once per cell cycle. *Genes Dev.* **14,** 2526–2533.

127. Nishitani, H., Taraviras, S., Lygerou, Z., and Nishimoto, T. (2001) The human licensing factor for DNA replication Cdt1 accumulates in G1 and is destabilized after initiation of S-phase. *JBC* **276,** 44905–44911.

128. Walter, J. C. (2000) Evidence for sequential action of Cdc7 and Cdk2 protein kinases during initiation of DNA replication in *Xenopus* egg extracts. *JBC* **275,** 39773–39778.

129. Walter, J. and Newport, J. (2000) Initiation of eukaryotic DNA replication: origin unwinding and sequential chromatin association of Cdc45, RPA, and DNA polymerase α. *Mol. Cell* **5,** 617–627.

130. Wohlschlegel, J. A., Dwyer, B. T., Dhar, S. K., Cvetic, C., Walter, J. C., and Dutta, A. (2000) Inhibition of eukaryotic DNA replication by geminin binding to Cdt1. *Science* **290,** 2309–2312.

131. Yanagi, K. I., Mizuno, T., You, Z., and Hanaoka, F. (2002) Mouse geminin inhibits not only Cdt1–MCM6 interactions but also a novel intrinsic Cdt1 DNA binding activity. *JBC* **277,** 40871–40880.

132. McGarry, T. J. (2002) Geminin deficiency causes a Chk1-dependent G2 arrest in *Xenopus. Mol. Cell. Biol.* **13,** 3662–3671.

133. McGarry, T. J. and Kirschner, M. W. (1998) Geminin, an inhibitor of DNA replication, is degraded during mitosis. *Cell* **93,** 1043–1053.

134. Yamaguchi, R. and Newport, J. (2003) A role for Ran-GTP and Crm1 in blocking re-replication. *Cell* **113,** 115–125.

135. Lee, J., Kumagai, A., and Dunphy, W. G. (2003) Claspin, a Chk1 regulatory protein, monitors DNA replication on chromatin independently of RPA, ATR, and Rad17. *Mol. Cell. Biol.* **11,** 329–340.

136. Zhao, H., Watkins, J. L., and Piwnica-Worms, H. (2002) Disruption of the checkpoint kinase 1/cell division cycle 25A pathway abrogates ionizing radiation–induced S and G2 checkpoints. *Proc. Nat. Acad. Sci. USA* **99,** 14795–14800.

137. Leone, G., Sears, R., Huang, E., et al. (2001) Myc requires distinct E2F activities to induce S phase and apoptosis. *Mol. Cell* **8,** 105–113.

138. Waga, S., Hannon, G. J., Beach, D., and Stillman, B. (1994) The p21 inhibitor of cyclin-dependent kinases controls DNA replication by interaction with PCNA. *Nature* **369,** 574–578.

139. Zhao, J., Dynlacht, B., Imai, T., Hori, T.-A., and Harlow, E. (1998) Expression of NPAT, a novel substrate of cyclin E–Cdk2, promotes S phase entry. *Genes Dev.* **12,** 456–461.

140. Elledge, S. J. (1996) Cell cycle checkpoints: preventing an identity crisis. *Science* **274,** 1664–1672.

141. Mailand, N., Podtelejnikov, A.V., Groth, A., Mann, M., Bartek, J., and Lukas, J. (2002) Regulation of G2/M events by Cdc25A through phosphorylation-dependent modulation of its stability. *EMBO J.* **21,** 5911–5920.

142. Dulic, V., Stein, G. H., Far, D. F., and Reed, S. J. (1998) Nuclear accumulation of p21 Cip1 at the onset of mitosis: a role at the G2/M phase transition. *Mol. Cell. Biol.* **18,** 546–557.

143. Hu, B., Mitra, J., Heuvel, S.V.D., and Enders, G. H. (2001) S and G2 phase role for Cdk2 revealed by inducible expression of a dominant-negative mutant in human cells. *Mol. Cell. Biol.* **21,** 2755–2766.

144. Clay-Farrace, L., Pelizon, C., Santamaria, D., Pines, J., and Laskey, R. A. (2003) Human replication protein Cdc6 prevents mitosis through a checkpoint mechanism that implicates Chk1. *EMBO J.* **22,** 704–712.

145. Musacchio, A. and Kardwick, K. G. (2002) The spindle checkpoint: structural insights into dynamic signaling. *Nat. Rev. Mol. Biol.* **3,** 731–741.

146. Russel, P. (1998) Checkpoints on the road to mitosis. *Trends Biochem. Sci.* **23,** 399–402.

147. Qian, Y. W., Erikson, E., Li, C., and Maller, J. L. (1998) Activated polo-like kinase Plx1 is required at multiple points during mitosis in *Xenopus laevis. Mol. Cell. Biol.* **18,** 4262–4271.

148. Kumagai, A. and Dunphy, W. G. (1996) Purification and molecular cloning of Plx1, a Cdc25-regulatory kinase from *Xenopus* egg extracts. *Science* **273,** 1377–1380.

149. Scolnick, D. M. and Halazonetis, T. D. (2000) Chfr defines a mitotic stress checkpoint that delays entry into metaphase. *Nature* **406,** 430–435.

150. Mollinari, C., Reynaud, C., Martineau-Thuillier, S., et al. (2003) The mammalian passenger protein TD-60 is an RC1 family member with an essential role in prometaphase to metaphase progression. *Dev. Cell* **5,** 295–307.

151. Cobbe, N. and Heck, M. M. (2000) SMCs in the world of chromosome biology—from prokaryotes to higher eukaryotes. *J. Struct. Biol.* **129,** 123–143.

152. Hirano, T. (2002) The ABCs of SMC proteins: two armed ATPpases for chromosome condensation, cohesion and repair. *Genes Dev.* **16,** 399–414.

153. Jessberger, R. (2001) The many functions of SMC proteins in chromosome dynamics. *Nat. Rev. Mol. Cell. Biol.* **3,** 767–778.

154. Hagstrom, K. A. and Meyer, B. J. (2003) Condensin and cohesin: more then chromosome compactor and glue. *Nat. Rev. Genet.* **4,** 520–534.

155. Gaucci, V., Koshland, D., and Strunnikov, A. (1997) A direct link between sister chromatid cohesion and chromosome condensation revealed through the analysis of MCD1 in *S. cerevisiae. Cell* **91,** 47–57.

156. Michalis, C., Ciosk, R., and Nasmyth, K. (1997) Cohesins: chromosomal proteins that prevent premature separation of sister chromatids. *Cell* **91,** 35–45.

158. Waizenegger, I. C., Hauf, S., Meinke, A., and Peters, J. M. (2000) Two distinct pathways remove mammalian cohesin from chromosome arms in prophase and from centromeres in anaphase. *Cell* **103,** 399–410.

159. Nasmyth, K. (2002) Segregating sister genomes: the molecular biology of chromosome separation. *Science* **297,** 559–565.

160. Peters, J. M. (2002) The anaphase-promoting complex: proteolysis in mitosis and beyond. *Mol. Cell* **9,** 931–943.

161. Hirano, T. and Mitchison, T. J. (1994) A heterodimeric coiled-coil protein required for mitotic chromosome condensation in vitro. *Cell* **79,** 449–458.

162. Hirano, T., Kobayashi, R., and Hirano, M. (1997) Condensins, chromosome condensation protein complexes containing XCAP-C, XCAP-E and a *Xenopus* homolog of the *Drosophila* Barren protein. *Cell* **89**, 511–521.

163. Musacchio, A. and Hardwick, K. G. (2002) The spindle checkpoint: structural insights into dynamic signaling. *Nat. Rev. Mol. Cell. Biol.* **3**, 731–741.

164. Hardwick, K. J. (1998) The spindle checkpoint. *Trends Genet.* **14**, 1–4.

164a. Hwang, L. H., Lau, L. F., Smith, D. L., et al. (1998) Budding yeast Cdc20: a target of the spindle checkpoint. *Science* **279**, 1041–1044.

164b. Kim, S. H., Lin, D. P., Matsumoto, S., Kitazono, A., and Matsumoto, T. (1998) Fission yeast Slp1: an effector of the Mad2-dependent spindle checkpoint. *Science* **279**, 1045–1047.

165. Maney, T., Ginkel, L. M., Hunter, A. W., and Wordeman, L. (2000) The kinetochores of higher eukaryotes: a molecular view. *Int. Rev. Cytol.* **194**, 67–131.

166. Chan, G. K. T., Schaar, B. T., and Yen, T. J. (1998) Characteization of the kinetochore binding domain of CENP-E reveals interactions with the kinetochore proteins CENP-F and hBUBR1. *J. Cell Biol.* **143**, 49–63.

167. Yao, X., Abrieu, A., Zheng, Y., Sullivan, K. F., and Cleveland, D. W. (2000) CENP-E forms a link between attachment of spindle microtubules and the mitotic checkpoint. *Nat. Cell Biol.* **2**, 484–491.

168. Abrieu, A., Kahana, J. A., Wood, K.W., and Cleveland, D. W. (2000) CENP-E as an essential component of the mitotic checkpoint in vitro. *Cell* **102**, 817–826.

169. Banks, J. D. and Heald, R. (2001) Chromosome movement: dynein-out at the kinetochore. *Curr. Biol.* **11**, R128–R131.

170. Starr, D. A., Williams, B. C., Hays, T. S., and Goldberg, M. L. (1998) ZW10 helps recruit dynactin and dynein to the kinetochores. *J. Cell Biol.* **142**, 763–774.

171. Chan, G. K., Jablonski, S. A., Starr, D. A., Goldberg, M. L., and Yen, T. J. (2000) Human Zw10 and ROD are mitotic checkpoint proteins that bind to kinetochores. *Nat. Cell Biol.* **2**, 939–943.

172. Chen, R. H. (2002) BubR1 is essential for kinetochore localization of other spindle checkpoint proteins and its phosphorylation requires Mad1. *J. Cell Biol.* **158**, 487–496.

173. Chen, R.-H., Waters, J. C., Salmon, E. D., and Murray, A. W. (1996) Association of spindle assembly checkpoint component XMAD2 with unattached kinetochores. *Science* **274**, 242–246.

174. Chen, R. H., Shevchenko, A., Mann, M., and Murray, A. W. (1998) Spindle checkpoint protein Xmad1 recruits Xmad2 to unattached kinetochores. *J. Cell Biol.* **143**, 283–295.

175. Chan, G. K., Schaar, B. T., and Yen, T. J. (1998) Characterization of the kinetochore binding domain of CENP-E reveals interactions with the kinetochore proteins CENP-E and hBUBR1. *J. Cell Biol.* **143**, 49–63.

176. Taylor, S. S. and McKeon, F. (1997) Kinetochore localization of murine Bub1 is required for normal mitotic timing and checkpoint response to spindle damage. *Cell* **89**, 727–735.

177. Taylor, S. S., Hussein, D., Wang, Y., Elderkin, S., and Morrow, C. J. (2001) Kinetochore localization and phosphorylation of the mitotic checkpoint compo-

211. Shou, W., Seol, J. H., Shevchenko, A. et al. (1999) Exit from mitosis is triggered by Tem1-dependent release of the protein phosphatase Cdc14 from nucleolar RENT complex. *Cell* **97**, 233–244.

212. Stegmeier, F., Visintin, R., and Amon, A. (2002) Separase, polo kinase, the kinetochore protein Slk19, and Spo12 function in a network that controls Cdc14 localization during early anaphase. *Cell* **108**, 207–220.

213. Jensen, S., Geymonat, M., and Johnston, L. H. (2002) Mitotic exit: delaying the end without FEAR. *Curr. Biol.* **12**, R221–R223.

214. Abrieu, A., Kahana, J. A., Wood, K. W., and Cleveland, D. W. (2000) CENP-E as an essential component of the mitotic checkpoint in vitro. *Cell* **102**, 817–826.

215. Kalab, P., Weis, K., and Heald, R. (2002) Visualization of Ran-GTP gradient in interphase and mitotic *Xenopus* egg extracts. *Science* **295**, 2452–2456.

216. Manser, E. (2002) Small GTPases take the stage. *Development* **3**, 323–328.

217. Walczak, C. E., Vernos, I., Mitchison, T. J., Karsenti, E., and Heald, R. (1998) Model for the proposed roles of different microtubule-based motor proteins in establishing spindle bipolarity. *Curr. Biol.* **8**, 903.

218. Walczak, C. E. (2001) Ran hits the ground running. *Nat. Cell. Biol.* **3**, E159–E161.

219. Sholey, J. M., Brust-Mascher, I., and Mogilner, A. (2003) Cell division. *Nature* **422**, 746–752.

220. Ohba, T., Nakamura, M., Nishitani, H., and Nishimoto, T. (1999) Self-organization of microtubule asters induced in *Xenopus* egg extracts by GTP-bound Ran. *Science* **284**, 1356–1358.

221. Gruss, O. J., Carazo-Salas, R. E., Schatz, C. A., Guarguaglini, G., Kast, J., Wilm, M., et al. (2001) Ran induces spindle assembly by reversing the inhibitory effect of importin α on TPX2 activity. *Cell* **104**, 83–93.

222. Terada, Y., Tatsuka, M., Suzuki, F., Yasuda, Y., Fujita, S., and Ostu, M. (1998) AIM-1: a mammalian midbody-associated protein required for cytokinesis. *EMBO J.* **17**, 667–676.

223. Hall, A. (1998) Rho GTPases and the actin cytoskeleton. *Science* **279**, 509–514.

224. Drechsel, D. N., Hyman, A. A., Hall, A., and Glotzer, M. (1997) A requirement for Rho and Cdc42 during cytokinesis in *Xenopus* embryos. *Curr. Biol.* **7**, 12–23.

225. Takaishi, K., Sasaki, T., Kato, M., et al. (1994) Involvement of Rho p21 small GTP-binding protein and its regulator in the HGF-induced cell motility. *Oncogene* **9**, 273–279.

226. Tatsumoto, T., Xie, X., Blumenthal, R., Okamoto, I., and Miki, T. (1999) Human ECT2 is an exchange factor for Rho GTPases, phosphorylated in G2/M phases, and involved in cytokinesis. *J. Cell Biol.* **147**, 921–928.

227. Hirose, K., Kawashima, T., Iwamoto, I., Nosaka, T., and Kitamura, T. (2001) MagRacGAP is involved in cytokinesis through associating with mitotic spindle and midbody. *JBC* **276**, 5821–5828.

228. Minoshima, Y., Kawashima, T., Hirose, K., et al. (2003) Phosphorylation by aurora B converts MgcRacGAP to a RhoGAP during cytokinesis. *Dev. Cell* **4**, 549–560.

229. Golsteyn, R. M., Mundt, K. E., Fry, A. M., and Nigg, E. A. (1995) Cell cycle regulation of the activity and subcellular localization of Plk1, a putative homolog of the mitotic spindle function. *J. Cell Biol.* **129**, 1617–1628.

230. Abraham, R. T. (2001) Cell cycle checkpoint signaling through the ATM and ATR kinases. *Genes Dev.* **15,** 2177–2196.
231. Bartek, J. and Lukas, J. (2001) Mammalian G1- and S-phase checkpoints in response to DNA damage. *Curr. Opin. Cell Biol.* **13,** 738–747.
232. Melo, J. and Toczski, D. (2002) A unified view of the DNA-damage checkpoint. *Curr. Opin. Cell Biol.* **14,** 237–245.
233. Shiloh, Y. (2003) ATM and related protein kinases: safeguarding genome integrity. *Nat. Rev. Cancer* **3,** 155–168.
234. Zhou, B. B. S. and Elledge, S. J. (2000) The DNA damage response: putting checkpoints in perspective. *Nature* **408,** 433–439.
235. McMahon, S. B., Wood, M. A., and Cole, M. D. (2000) The essential cofactor TRRAP recruits the histone acetylase hGCN5 to c-Myc. *Mol. Cell. Biol.* **20,** 556–562.
236. Durocher, D. and Jackson, S. P. (2001) DNA-PK, ATM and ATR as sensors of DNA damage: variations on a theme? *Curr. Opin. Cell Biol.* **13,** 225–231.
237. Edwards, R. J., Bentley, N. J., and Carr, A. M. (1999) A Rad3–Rad26 complex responds to DNA damage independently of other checkpoint proteins. *Nat. Cell Biol.* **1,** 393–398.
238. Cortez, D., Guntuku, S., Qin, J., and Elledge, S. J. (2001) ATR and ATRIP: parents in checkpoint signaling. *Science* **294,** 1713–1716.
239. Wakayama, T., Kondo, T., Ando, S., Matsumoto, K., and Sugimoto, K. (2001) Pie1, a protein interacting with Mex1, controls cell growth and checkpoint responses in *Saccharomyces cerevisiae. Mol. Cell. Biol.* **21,** 755–764.
240. Melo, J. A., Cohen, J., and Toczyski, D. P. (2001) Two checkpoint complexes are independently recruited to sites of DNA damage in vivo. *Genes Dev.* **15,** 2809–2821.
241. Costanzo, V., Robertson, K., Ying, C. Y., et al. (2000) Reconstitution of an ATM-dependent checkpoint that inhibits chromosomal DNA replication following DNA damage. *Mol. Cell* **6,** 649–659.
242. Smith, G. C., Cary, R. B., Lakin, N. D., et al. (1999) Purification of DNA binding properties of the ataxia-telangiectasia gene product ATM. *Proc. Nat. Acad. Sci. USA* **96,** 11134–11139.
243. Andegeko, Y., Moyal, L., Mittelman, L., Tsarfaty, I., Shiloh, Y., and Rotman, G. (2001) Nuclear retention of ATM at sites of DNA double strand break. *JBC* **276,** 38224–38230.
244. Bakkenist, C. J. and Kastan, M. B. (2003) DNA damage activates ATM through intermolecular autophosphorylation and dimer dissociation. *Nature* **42,** 499–506.
245. Petrini, J. H. (2000) The Mre11 complex and ATM: collaborating to navigate S phase checkpoint regulations. *Genes Dev.* **15,** 2238–2249.
246. Lim, D. S., Kim, S. T., Xu, B., Maser, R. S., Lin, J., Petrini, J. H., et al. (2000) ATM phosphorylates p95/nbs1 in an S-phase checkpoint pathway. *Nature* **404,** 613–617.
247. Zhao, S., Weng, Y. C., Yuan, S. S., Lin, Y.T., Hsu, H.C., Lin, S. C., et al. (2000) Functional link between ataxia-telangiectasia and Nijmegen breakage syndrome gene products. *Nature* **405,** 473–477.

352. Zeng, Y., Forbes, C. K., Wu, Z., Moreno, S., Piwnica-Worms, H., and Enoch, T. (1998) Replication checkpoint requires phosphorylation of the phosphatase Cdc25 by Cds1 or Chk1. *Nature* **395,** 507–510.

353. Hoffmann, I., Draetta, G., and Karsenti, E. (1994) Activation of the phosphatase activity of human cdc25A by a cdk2-cyclin E dependent phosphorylation at the G1/S transition. *EMBO J.* **13,** 4302–4310.

354. Xiao, Z, Chen, Z., Gunasekera, A. H., et al. (2003) Chk1 mediates S and G2 arrests through Cdc25A degradation in response to DNA-damaging agents. *JBC* **278,** 21767–21773.

354. Karlsson, C., Katich, S., Hagting, A., Hoffman, I., and Pines, J. (1999) Cdc25B and Cdc25C differ markedly in their properties as initiators of mitosis. *J. Cell Biol.* **146,** 573–584.

355. Peng, C.-Y., Graves, P. R., Thoma, R. S., Wu, Z., Shaw, A. S., and Piwnica-Worms, H. (1997) Mitotic and G2 checkpoint control: regulation of 14-3-3 protein binding by phosphorylation of Cdc25C on serine-216. *Science* **277,** 1501–1505.

356. Sanchez, Y. Wong, C., Thoma, R. S., et al. (1997) Conservation of the Chk1 checkpoint pathway in mammals: linkage of DNA damage to Cdk regulation through Cdc25C. *Science* **277,** 1497–1501.

357. Lopez-Girona, A., Furnari, B., Mondesert, O., and Russell, P. (1999) Nuclear localization of Cdc25 is regulated by DNA damage and a 14-3-3 protein. *Nature* **397,** 172–175

358. Furnari, B., Blasina, A., Boddy, M. N., McGowan, C. H., and Russell, P. (1999) Cdc25 inhibited in vivo and in vitro by checkpoint kinases cds1 and chk1. *Mol. Cell Biol.* **10,** 833–845.

359. Weinert, T. A. (1997) DNA damage checkpoint meets the cell cycle engine. *Science* **277,** 1450–1451.

360. Xu, B., Kim, S., and Kastan, M. B. (2001) Involvement of Brca1 in S-phase and G2-phase checkpoints after ionizing irradiation. *Mol. Cell Biol.* **21,** 3445–3450.

361. Xu, X., Weaver, Z., Linke, S. P., et al. (1999) Centrosome amplification and a defective G2-M cell cycle checkpoint induce genetic instability in BRCA1 exon 11 isoform-deficient cells. *Mol. Cell* **3,** 389–395.

362. Cheng, I., Hunke, I., and Hardy, C. (1998) Cell cycle regulation of the *Saccharomyces cerevisiae* polo-like kinase Cdc5p. *Mol. Cell Biol.* **18,** 7360–7370.

363. Sanchez, Y., Bachant, J., Wang, H., et al. (1999) Control of the DNA damage checkpoint by Chk1 and Rad53 protein kinases through distinct mechanisms. *Science* **286,** 1166–1171.

364. Qian, Y. W., Erikson, E., Li, C., and Maller, J. I. (1998) Activated polo-like kinase Plx1 is required at multiple points during mitosis in *Xenopus laevis. Mol. Cell Biol.* **18,** 4262–4271.

365. Smits, V. A., Klompmaker, R., Arnaud, L., Rijksen, G., Nigg, E. A., and Medema, R. H. (2000) Polo-like kinase-1 is a target of the DNA damage checkpoint. *Nat. Cell Biol.* **2,** 672–676.

366. Malumbres, M. and Barbacid, M. (2001) To cycle or not to cycle: a critical decision in cancer. *Nat. Rev. Cancer* **1,** 222–231.

367. Hall, M. and Peters, G. (1996) Genetic alterations of cyclins, cyclin-dependent kinases, and Cdk inhibitors in human cancer. *Adv. Cancer Res.* **68,** 67–108.

368. Loda, M., Cukor, B., Tam, S. W., et al. (1997) Increased proteosome-dependent degradation of the cyclin-dependent kinase inhibitor p27 in aggressive colorectal carcinomas. *Nat. Med.* **3,** 231–234.

369. Bell, D. W., Varley, J. M., Szydlo, T. E., et al. (1999) Heterozygous germ line hCHK2 mutations in Lifraumeni syndrome. *Science* **286,** 2528–2531.

370. Jin, D. Y., Spencer, F., and Jeang, K. T. (1998) Human T cell leukemia virus type 1 oncoprotein Tax targets the human mitotic checkpoint protein MAD1. *Cell* **93,** 81–91.

371. Zou, H., McGarry, T. J., Bernal, T., and Kirschner, M. W. (1999) Identification of a vertebrate sister-chromatid separation inhibitor involved in transformation and tumorigenesis. *Science* **285,** 418–422.

372. Gemma, A., Seike, M., Seike, Y., et al. (2000) Somatic mutations of the hBUB1 mitotic checkpoint gene in primary lung cancer. *Genes Chromo. Can.* **29,** 213–218.

373. Cahill, D. P., Lengauer, C., Yu, J., et al. (1998) Mutations of mitotic checkpoint genes in human cancer. *Nature* **392,** 300– 303.

374. Reis, R. M., Nakamura, M., Masuoka, J., et al. (2001) Mitotic checkpoint genes hBUB1, hBUB1B, hBUB3 and TTK in human bladder cancer, screening for mutations and loss of heterozygosity. *Carcinogenesis* **22,** 813–815.

375. Wu , C., Kinrley, S. D., Xial, H., Chung, Y., Chung, D. C., and Zukerberg, L. R. (2001) Cables enhances Cdk2 tyrosine 15 phosphorylation by Wee1, inhibits cell growth, and is lost in many human colon and squamous cancers. *Cancer Res.* **61,** 7325–7332.

376. Corn, P. G., Summers, M. K., Fogt, F., et al. (2003) Frequent hypermethylation of the 5' CpG island of the mitotic stress checkpoint gene Chfr in colorectal and non-small cell lung cancer. *Carcinogenesis* **24,** 47–51.

II

ANALYZING CHECKPOINT CONTROLS IN DIVERSE MODEL SYSTEMS

5

Establishment of a Cell-Free System to Study the Activation of Chk2

Xingzhi Xu and David F. Stern

Summary

The checkpoint kinase Chk2 is activated in response to DNA damage through pathways requiring protein kinases ATM and/or ATR. The means by which Chk2 is activated by these kinases still remains to be addressed. Here we describe a cell-free system to study the activation of Chk2. Chk2 produced by a wheat germ extract in vitro transcription/translation system is inactive and can be activated by incubating with a rabbit reticulocyte lysate. This method will be useful for identification of cofactors required for activation of Chk2.

Key Words: Checkpoint kinase; Chk2; kinase assay; ataxia telangiectasia mutated (ATM); DNA damage; in vitro translation; wheat germ extract; reticulocyte lysate.

1. Introduction

The checkpoint kinase Chk2 is an evolutionarily conserved serine/threonine kinase. Chk2 has an amino-terminal SQ/TQ cluster domain (SCD), followed by a forkhead-associated (FHA) domain and a carboxyl-terminal kinase catalytic domain *(1–3)*. In response to ionizing radiation (IR) and other DNA double-stranded break (DSB)-producing agents, Chk2 is rapidly phosphorylated at Thr 68 and other SQ/TQ sites within the SCD by the phospho-inositide kinase related kinase (PIKK) ATM (ataxia telangiectasia mutated) *(4–7)*. Priming phosphorylation at Thr 68 by ATM is required, but not sufficient, for Chk2 activation. This priming phosphorylation may promote Chk2 oligomerization, intermolecular cross-phosphorylation, and then full activation *(8,9)*. In budding yeast, the ATM/ATR (ATM and Rad3-related) ortholog Mec1 is a master regulator of cellular responses to DNA damage. In response to DNA damage, Rad9 is phosphorylated in a *MEC1*-dependent manner *(10–12)* and, in turn, phosphorylated Rad9 apparently recruits the Chk2 ortholog Rad53 *(13,14)* to

From: *Methods in Molecular Biology, vol. 280: Checkpoint Controls and Cancer, Volume 1: Reviews and Model Systems*
Edited by: Axel H. Schönthal © Humana Press Inc., Totowa, NJ

the Mec1 complex for activation. (Note that budding yeast Rad9 is unrelated to human RAD9.) Alternatively, phosphorylated Rad9 oligomers may act as a scaffold to bring Rad53 molecules into close proximity to each other, facilitating cross-phosphorylation between Rad53 molecules and subsequent release of activated Rad53 *(15)*. Rad9 also regulates activation of Chk1, another important effector kinase of Mec1, in the G2/M checkpoint *(16)*. BRCA1 *(17)*, 53BP1 *(18–22)*, and MDC1 (mediator of DNA damage checkpoint protein 1)/ NFBD1/KIAA0170 *(23–29)* are candidate RAD9 orthologs in mammals. Substrates for Chk2 include p53 *(30–32)*, Brca1 *(33)*, Cdc25A *(34)*, and Cdc25C *(1–3,35)*. Phosphorylation of these substrates by Chk2 contributes to IR-induced cell cycle arrest and apoptosis. However, the means by which Chk2 is activated by ATM still remains to be addressed. Efforts to activate mammalian Chk2 in vitro by phosphorylation with ATM *(5)* or the PIKK DNA-PK (DNA-dependent protein kinase) *(8)* have been unsuccessful. We have established the first mammalian cell-free system to enable catalytic activation of Chk2 *(8)*. This will be a useful tool for identification of cofactors required for the ATM-dependent activation of Chk2.

2. Materials

1. Plasmids: A clone within the expressed sequence tag (EST) database (GenBank accession no. AA285249) containing the entire coding sequence of Chk2 was obtained from the Wistar Institute (courtesy of Thanos D. Halazonetis).
2. Primers: T7: 5' taa tac gac tca cta tag gg 3'. CDNA.R: 5' att tag gtg aca cta tag aa 3'. D347A.S: 5' gaa aac ggt att ata cac cgt g<u>c</u>c tta aag cca gag aat gtt tta ctg3'; the underlined nucleotide is A in wild-type Chk2. R, reverse primer; S, sense primer.
3. High-fidelity DNA polymerase, Pwo (Roche Molecular Biochemicals).
4. $T_N T^\circledR$ T7 quick-coupled transcription/translation system (Promega). This system is supplied with $T_N T^\circledR$ quick master mix, 1 mM methionine, and nuclease-free water.
5. $T_N T^\circledR$ T7 coupled wheat germ extract system (Promega). *This system is supplied with $T_N T^\circledR$ wheat germ extract, $T_N T^\circledR$ T7 RNA polymerase, $T_N T^\circledR$ reaction buffer (25X), and amino acid mixture minus methionine.*
6. RNasin ribonuclease inhibitor (Roche Molecular Biochemicals).
7. Antibodies: Rabbit polyclonal anti-T26/S28 or anti-T68 Chk2 antibodies are commercially available from Cell Signaling Technology. Mouse monoclonal anti-HA antibody (clone 16B12) is from Covance. Horseradish peroxidase (HRP)-conjugated rat anti-HA (clone 3F10) monoclonal antibodies are from Roche. Antigen–antibody complexes are recovered with protein G plus protein A agarose (CalBiochem). HRP-conjugated secondary antibodies and chemiluminescent reagents are from Pierce.
8. Protease inhibitor cocktail (Roche Molecular Biochemicals).

9. NETN buffer: 20 m*M* Tris-HCl, pH 8.0, 0.1 *M* NaCl, 1 m*M* EDTA, 0.5% NP-40, and protease inhibitor cocktail. NETN buffer lacking protease inhibitor cocktail is stored at 4°C. Protease inhibitor cocktail is added to the buffer fresh.
10. 2X kinase buffer: 40 m*M* Tris-HCl, pH 7.5, 20 m*M* MgCl$_2$, 20 m*M* MnCl$_2$, 2 m*M* DTT.
11. [γ-^{32}P] ATP (>5000 Ci/mmol, AA0018, Amersham Pharmacia Biotech).
12. ATP (10 m*M*, Promega): Stock solution is diluted to a final concentration of 100 μ*M* in H$_2$O. Both stock and diluted solutions are stored in aliquots in –70°C freezer. Repeated freeze and thaw should be avoided.
13. PBS-T buffer: phosphate-buffered saline (0.2 g/L KCl, 0.2 g/L CaCl$_2$, 8 g/L NaCl, and 2.16 g/L Na$_2$HPO$_4$·7H$_2$O) with 0.05% Tween-20.
14. Sodium dodecyl sulfate-polyacrylamide gel eletrophoresis (SDS-PAGE) equipment.
15. SDS sample buffer: 62.5 m*M* Tris-HCl, pH 6.8, 20% glycerol, 2% SDS, 5% β-mercaptoethanol.
16. Semi-dry immunoblot transfer equipment (BioRad).
17. Nitrocellulose membrane (0.2 μm, BioRad).
18. Benchtop cooler.

3. Methods

The methods described below outline (1) the construction of the expression plasmids; (2) in vitro coupled transcription/translation assays; (3) immunoprecipitations; (4) in vitro kinase assays; (5) activation of Chk2 produced in the wheat germ extract system; and (6) immunoblotting and monitoring ^{32}P incorporation.

3.1. Expression Constructs

3.1.1. Mammalian Expression Vector

pcDNA3HA (the parental plasmid pcDNA3 is from Invitrogen) is a mammalian expression vector under the control of a human cytomegalovirus (CMV) immediate-early promoter with an amino-terminal tag consisting of three copies of the HA epitope. A T7 promoter/priming site is located between the CMV promoter and the HA epitope tag. This allows for in vitro transcription in the sense orientation and sequencing through the insert. The primer CDNA.R is complementary to a region that is downstream of the multiple cloning sites of this vector.

3.1.2. Wild-Type Chk2

Chk2-coding sequences were amplified by polymerase chain reaction (PCR) from the Chk2 EST clone, and cloned into the EcoRI site of pcDNA3HA, resulting in pcDNA-HAChk2.

3.1.3. Kinase-Defective Chk2

Kinase-defective Chk2 was generated from pcDNA-HAChk2 using PCR-based site-directed mutagenesis *(36)*. We mutated sequences encoding the conserved aspartic acid residue at 347 within the ATP binding pocket to encode alanine. On the template of pcDNA-HAChk2, the combination of the primers CDNA.R and D347A.S amplified a fragment of approximately 700 bp. This resulting fragment, in combination with T7 primer, amplified a fragment of approx 1.7 kbp on the template of pcDNA-HAChk2. This final PCR product, which contained the point mutation, was digested with EcoRI and cloned into the EcoRI site of pcDNA3xHA, resulting in pcDNA-HAChk2(D347A).

The authenticity of the cloned sequences was confirmed by sequencing. The kinase activity of both wild-type and kinase-defective Chk2 was determined by in vitro kinase assays (*see* **Note 1**).

3.2. In Vitro Coupled Transcription/Translation Assays

The Chk2 constructs (both wild-type and kinase-defective) are used as templates for in vitro transcription/translation of Chk2. Promega $T_NT^®$ T7 Quick Coupled Transcription/Translation reticulocyte lysate system and T7 Coupled Transcription/Translation wheat germ extract system are used according to procedures recommended by the manufacturer (*see* **Note 2**).

3.2.1. Chk2 Produced in the Rabbit Reticulocyte Lysate System

1. Rapidly thaw the $T_NT^®$ quick master mix by hand warming and then place on ice. The other components are thawed at room temperature and then kept on ice.
2. Mix the following components on ice in a sterile 1.5 mL microcentrifuge tube: 40 μL of $T_NT^®$ quick master mix, 2 μL of plasmid DNA template (pcDNA-HA vector, pcDNA-HAChk2, or pcDNA-HAChk2[D347A]) at a concentration of 0.5 μg/μL, 7 μL of nuclease-free water, and 1 μL of 1 mM methionine.
3. Incubate the reaction at 30°C for 90 min (*see* **Notes 3** and **4**).

3.2.2. Chk2 Produced in the Wheat Germ Extract System

1. Rapidly thaw the $T_NT^®$ wheat germ extract by hand warming and then place on ice. Keep the $T_NT^®$ T7 RNA polymerase in a benchtop cooler. Allow other components to thaw at room temperature and then store on ice.
2. Mix the following components on ice in a sterile 1.5 mL microcentrifuge tube: 25 μL of $T_NT^®$ wheat germ extract, 2 μL of 25X $T_NT^®$ reaction buffer, 4 μL of plasmid DNA template (pcDNA-HAChk2 or pcDNA-HAChk2(D347A) (*see* **Note 5**) at the concentration of 0.5 μg/μL, 15 μL of nuclease-free water, 1 μL of RNasin ribonuclease inhibitor, 1 μL of amino acid mixture minus methionine, 1 μL of 1 mM methionine, and 1 μL of $T_NT^®$ T7 RNA polymerase.
3. Incubate the reaction at 30°C for 2 h (*see* **Notes 3** and **4**).

3.3. Immunoprecipitations

1. Combine the in vitro translation product (8 μL from the rabbit reticulocyte lysate system or 15 μL from the wheat germ extract system) with 300 μL of NETN buffer.
2. Add 2 μg of anti-HA antibody (clone 16B12) to each sample and incubate on a roller at 4°C for 3 h.
3. Add 20 μL of 50% protein G plus protein A agarose slurry in PBS to each sample and incubate on a roller at 4°C for an additional hour (*see* **Note 6**).
4. Collect immune complexes by centrifugation at a speed of 5000*g* for 1 min in a refrigerated microcentrifuge.
5. Wash precipitates three times by inverting the tubes several times with approx 1.5 mL of NETN buffer lacking protease inhibitors. Collect immune complexes as described in **step 4**.
6. Further wash immune complexes twice in approx 1.5 mL of 1X kinase buffer.
7. Keep tubes with pellet on ice until next step.

3.4. In Vitro Kinase Assays

1. Prepare a master reaction mixture: each 50-μL reaction contains 25 μL of 2X kinase buffer, 1 μL of 100 μ*M* nonlabeled ATP and 10 μCi of [γ-^{32}P]ATP (*see* **Note 7**).
2. Add 50 μL reaction mix to purified immunocomplexes (from **Subheading 3.7., step 3.**) and incubate at 30°C for 5–10 min, intermittently tapping the tubes two to three times.
3. Terminate kinase reaction by adding 50 μL of SDS sample buffer.
4. Boil 5 min at 95°C and keep ready for SDS-PAGE. For long-term storage (up to 2 wk), keep samples in –20°C freezer.

3.5. Activation of Chk2 Produced in the Wheat Germ Extract System

1. Add 20 μL of T$_N$T® quick master mix from the reticulocyte lysate system to the immune complexes in **Subheading 3.3., step 7**, derived from the wheat germ extract system.
2. Incubate the mixture at 30°C for 30 min, intermittently tapping the tubes three to four times.
3. Wash the immune complex three times in NETN buffer and then twice in 1X kinase buffer as described in **Subheading 3.3., steps 4–7.**.
4. Perform in vitro kinase assays as described in **Subheading 3.4.**

3.6. Immunoblotting and Monitoring ^{32}P Incorporation

1. Resolve the kinase assay products derived from **Subheadings 3.4.** and **3.5.** on an 8% SDS-PAGE (acrylamide:bisacrylamide is 37.5:1) and transfer to a nitrocellulose membrane using a BioRad semi-dry blotting system at 15 V for 42 min (*see* **Notes 2** and **8**).

3. Matsuoka, S., Huang, M., and Elledge, S. J. (1998) Linkage of ATM to cell cycle regulation by the Chk2 protein kinase. *Science* **282**, 1893–1897.
4. Ahn, J. Y., Schwarz, J. K., Piwnica-Worms, H., and Canman, C. E. (2000) Threonine 68 phosphorylation by ataxia telangiectasia mutated is required for efficient activation of Chk2 in response to ionizing radiation. *Cancer Res.* **60**, 5934–5936.
5. Matsuoka, S., Rotman, G., Ogawa, A., Shiloh, Y., Tamai, K., and Elledge, S. J. (2000) Ataxia telangiectasia-mutated phosphorylates Chk2 in vivo and in vitro. *Proc. Natl. Acad. Sci. USA* **97**, 10389–10394.
6. Melchionna, R., Chen, X. B., Blasina, A., and McGowan, C. H. (2000) Threonine 68 is required for radiation-induced phosphorylation and activation of Cds1. *Nat. Cell Biol.* **2**, 762–765.
7. Zhou, B. B., Chaturvedi, P., Spring, K., et al. (2000) Caffeine abolishes the mammalian G(2)/M DNA damage checkpoint by inhibiting ataxia-telangiectasia-mutated kinase activity. *J. Biol. Chem.* **275**, 10342–10348.
8. Xu, X., Tsvetkov, L. M., and Stern, D. F. (2002) Chk2 activation and phosphorylation-dependent oligomerization. *Mol. Cell. Biol.* **22**, 4419–4432.
9. Ahn, J. Y., Li, X., Davis, H. L., and Canman, C. E. (2002) Phosphorylation of threonine 68 promotes oligomerization and autophosphorylation of the Chk2 protein kinase via the forkhead-associated domain. *J. Biol. Chem.* **277**, 19,389–19,395.
10. Emili, A. (1998) MEC1-dependent phosphorylation of Rad9p in response to DNA damage. *Mol. Cell* **2**, 183–189.
11. Sun, Z., Fay, D. S., Marini, F., Foiani, M., and Stern, D. F. (1996) Spk1/Rad53 is regulated by Mec1-dependent protein phosphorylation in DNA replication and damage checkpoint pathways. *Genes Dev.* **10**, 395–406.
12. Sanchez, Y., Desany, B. A., Jones, W. J., Liu, Q., Wang, B., and Elledge, S. J. (1996) Regulation of RAD53 by the ATM-like kinases MEC1 and TEL1 in yeast cell cycle checkpoint pathways. *Science* **271**, 357–360.
13. Sun, Z., Hsiao, J., Fay, D. S., and Stern, D. F. (1998) Rad53 FHA domain associated with phosphorylated Rad9 in the DNA damage checkpoint. *Science* **281**, 272–274.
14. Vialard, J. E., Gilbert, C. S., Green, C. M., and Lowndes, N. F. (1998) The budding yeast Rad9 checkpoint protein is subjected to Mec1/Tel1-dependent hyperphosphorylation and interacts with Rad53 after DNA damage. *EMBO J.* **17**, 5679–5688.
15. Gilbert, C. S., Green, C. M., and Lowndes, N. F. (2001) Budding yeast Rad9 is an ATP-dependent Rad53 activating machine. *Mol. Cell* **8**, 129–136.
16. Sanchez, Y., Bachant, J., Wang, H., et al. (1999) Control of the DNA damage checkpoint by chk1 and rad53 protein kinases through distinct mechanisms. *Science* **286**, 1166–1171.
17. Yarden, R. I., Pardo-Reoyo, S., Sgagias, M., Cowan, K. H., and Brody, L. C. (2002) BRCA1 regulates the G2/M checkpoint by activating Chk1 kinase upon DNA damage. *Nat. Genet.* **30**, 285–289.
18. Schultz, L. B., Chehab, N. H., Malikzay, A., and Halazonetis, T. D. (2000) p53 binding protein 1 (53BP1) is an early participant in the cellular response to DNA double-strand breaks. *J. Cell Biol.* **151**, 1381–1390.

19. Rappold, I., Iwabuchi, K., Date, T., and Chen, J. (2001) Tumor suppressor p53 binding protein 1 (53BP1) is involved in DNA damage-signaling pathways. *J. Cell Biol.* **153,** 613–620.

20. Anderson, L., Henderson, C., and Adachi, Y. (2001) Phosphorylation and rapid relocalization of 53BP1 to nuclear foci upon DNA damage. *Mol. Cell. Biol.* **21,** 1719–1729.

21. Wang, B., Matsuoka, S., Carpenter, P. B., and Elledge, S. J. (2002) 53BP1, a mediator of the DNA damage checkpoint. *Science* **298,** 1435–1438.

22. DiTullio, R. A., Jr., Mochan, T. A., Venere, M., et al. (2002) 53BP1 functions in an ATM-dependent checkpoint pathway that is constitutively activated in human cancer. *Nat. Cell Biol.* **4,** 998–1002.

23. Goldberg, M., Stucki, M., Falck, J., et al. (2003) MDC1 is required for the intra-S-phase DNA damage checkpoint. *Nature* **421,** 952–956.

24. Lou, Z., Minter-Dykhouse, K., Wu, X., and Chen, J. (2003) MDC1 is coupled to activated CHK2 in mammalian DNA damage response pathways. *Nature* **421,** 957–961.

25. Peng, A. and Chen, P. L. (2003) NFBD1, like 53BP1, is an early and redundant transducer mediating Chk2 phosphorylation in response to DNA damage. *J. Biol. Chem.* **278,** 8873–8876.

26. Shang, Y. L., Bodero, A. J., and Chen, P. L. (2003) NFBD1, a novel nuclear protein with signature motifs of FHA and BRCT, and an internal 41-amino acid repeat sequence, is an early participant in DNA damage response. *J. Biol. Chem.* **278,** 6323–6329.

27. Stewart, G. S., Wang, B., Bignell, C. R., Taylor, A. M., and Elledge, S. J. (2003) MDC1 is a mediator of the mammalian DNA damage checkpoint. *Nature* **421,** 961–966.

28. Xu, X. and Stern, D. F. (2003) NFBD1/KIAA0170 is a chromatin-associated protein involved in DNA damage signaling pathways. *J. Biol. Chem.* **278,** 8795–8803.

29. Xu, X. and Stern, D. F. (2003) NFBD1/MDC1 regulates ionizing radiation–induced focus formation of DNA checkpoint signaling and repair factors. *FASEB J.* 18,1842–1848.

30. Chehab, N. H., Malikzay, A., Appel, M., and Halazonetis, T. D. (2000) Chk2/hCds1 functions as a DNA damage checkpoint in G(1) by stabilizing p53. *Genes Dev.* **14,** 278–288.

31. Hirao, A., Kong, Y. Y., Matsuoka, S., et al. (2000) DNA damage–induced activation of p53 by the checkpoint kinase Chk2. *Science* **287,** 1824–1827.

32. Shieh, S. Y., Ahn, J., Tamai, K., Taya, Y., and Prives, C. (2000) The human homologs of checkpoint kinases Chk1 and Cds1 (Chk2) phosphorylate p53 at multiple DNA damage–inducible sites. *Genes Dev.* **14,** 289–300.

33. Lee, J. S., Collins, K. M., Brown, A. L., Lee, C. H., and Chung, J. H. (2000) hCds1-mediated phosphorylation of BRCA1 regulates the DNA damage response. *Nature* **404,** 201–204.

34. Falck, J., Mailand, N., Syljuasen, R. G., Bartek, J., and Lukas, J. (2001) The ATM–Chk2–Cdc25A checkpoint pathway guards against radioresistant DNA synthesis. *Nature* **410,** 842–847.

cells, particularly the stem cells in the basal layer of the skin *(2–4)*. The cell cycle response observed is different from that observed with in vitro cultured primary melanocytes and keratinocytes, suggesting that the tissue microenvironment influences cell cycle responses of the basal layer cells.

2. Materials

1. RPMI 1640 medium (Gibco BRL), supplemented with 10% donor calf serum (Serum Supreme, Biowhittaker), penicillin/streptomycin liquid (100X) (Gibco BRL containing 10,000 U/mL penicillin G and 10,000 μg/mL streptomycin sulfate), garamycin (100X stock concentration of 40 mg/mL), and fungizone (5 mg/mL 1,000X stock solution; Apthecon).
2. MCDB153 medium (Sigma) containing penicillin/streptomycin and fungizone as in **item 1**.
3. Sodium hypochlorite (100 g/L available chlorine).
4. Versene: 18.5 g NaCl, 0.4 g KCl, 2.3 g Na_2HPO_4, 0.4 g KH_2PO_4, 4.52 g EDTA (tetrasodium salt); make up to 2 L using MilliQ 4 grade water. Autoclave to sterilize.
5. HEPES (1 *M*): 238.0 g HEPES; make up to 1 L using MilliQ 4 grade water. Autoclave to sterilize.
6. Phosphate buffered saline, sterile (PBS): 8.5 g NaCl, 1.48 g Na_2HPO_4, 0.43 g KH_2PO_4; make up to 1 L using MilliQ 4 grade water. Autoclave to sterilize. Sterile instruments: scissors, fine-nose forceps, scalpel handle (no. 4), scalpel blade (no. 22).
7. 5-bromo-2'-deoxyuridine (BrdU) (ICN): prepared as a 500 m*M* stock dissolved in DMSO.
8. BioRad DC (Detergent Compatible) Protein Assay.
9. Histostain-DS kit (Zymed Laboratories Inc., Cat. No. 95-9999).
10. Double Stain Enhancer (Zymed Laboratories Inc., Cat. No. 50-506).
11. Collection medium: 90 mL RPMI 1640 medium, 10 mL serum supreme, 300 μL HEPES, 100 μL penicillin/streptomycin solution, 100 μL garamycin, 100 μL fungizone. Aliquot 5 mL into sterile tubes.
12. Culturing medium: 1 L MCDB153 medium, 1 mL penicillin/streptomycin liquid, 1 mL fungizone.
13. Lysis buffer (NETN): 100 m*M* NaCl, 1 m*M* EDTA, 0.5% Nonidet P-40, 20 m*M* Tris -HCl pH 8.00 supplemented with 200 m*M* NaCl, 5 μg/mL aprotinin, 5 μg/mL leupeptin, 5 μg/mL pepstatin, 10 m*M* NaF, 0.1 m*M* sodium orthovanadate, 0.5 m*M* phenylmethylsulphonyl fluoride (PMSF), added immediately prior to use.
14. Polytron tissue homogenizer, model PT1200C, with 7.5 mm aggregate (Kinematica AG, Switzerland).
15. Ultracentrifuge, Beckman TL-100 (Beckman).

3. Methods

The collection and preparation of foreskin tissue has been optimized to maintain tissue viability and integrity. It is essential that tissue samples be collected and processed with minimal delay and in a manner that does not subject the tissue to any physical trauma, which may adversely affect subsequent analyses.

3.1. Collection of Tissue and Preparation of Organ Cultures

Neonatal foreskins are immersed in 5–10 mL of cold collection medium immediately following surgery and are maintained at 4°C during transport (*see* **Note 1**). To prepare the foreskin tissue for organ culture, the tissue is processed to minimize any risk of bacterial or fungal contamination during subsequent culturing. For all subsequent manipulation, foreskins are handled by gently grasping the very edge of the specimen with forceps.

1. Immerse foreskin in 10 mL sodium hypochlorite for approx 1–2 min to reduce the possibility of fungal contamination. Shake gently.
2. Immerse foreskin in Versene for approx 1–2 min to remove red blood cells and neutralize hypochlorite. Swirl gently.
3. Wash twice with 30 mL sterile PBS with gentle swirling for 1–2 min.
4. Immerse in 50 mL sterile PBS.
5. Place in 10-cm Petri dish, and remove as much subcutaneous fatty tissue as possible, ensuring not to damage the tissue by pulling and prodding. Place the tissue with the epidermis facing downwards, and use fine-nose forceps to grasp a small amount of tissue from the center of the subcutaneous fatty tissue. Use very sharp sterile scissors to cut away small amounts of fatty tissue. Repeat the procedure by picking up small areas of fatty tissue with the forceps, and cutting just below the forceps with scissors. It is extremely important that the tissue be treated in a very gentle manner, and that the tissue not undergo any trauma as a result of trimming the subcutaneous fatty tissue. Removal of this subcutaneous fatty tissue from along the length of the dermal side of the foreskin will enable the skin to lie flat in the Petri dish (*see* **Note 2**).
6. Briefly rinse in PBS.
7. Place the tissue in a 5-cm petri dish with the epidermis facing upwards, and add MCDB153 culturing medium until the foreskin tissue appears to float on top of the medium. The epidermis should remain exposed to the air-liquid interface.
8. Maintain at 37°C and 5% CO_2 in a tissue-culture incubator and change medium on a daily basis.

3.2. Treatment of Organ Cultures

Organ cultures afford the opportunity to perform various manipulations and detailed analysis of cell cycle progression using techniques usually restricted to cultured cell lines for human studies. For example, the foreskins can be treated with a range of soluble agents, such as growth factors and mitogens, or cells can be labeled using 5-bromo-2'-deoxyuridine (BrdU) to identify those cells that have passed into S phase during the course of the experiment.

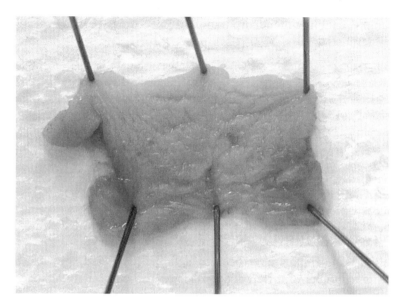

Fig. 1. After harvesting, the foreskin is pinned to a piece of foam before fixing.

Note 6). It is essential that the fixation times remain constant between samples, and that all samples be handled in a consistent manner.

3. Prior to paraffin embedding, cut the tissue into longitudinal slices, which will enable a number of faces of the epidermis to be visualized within each section (*see* **Note 7**).

4. Process the tissue using standard protocols for paraffin embedding. Samples for light microscopy and immunohistochemistry were processed using a Shandon Hypercenter XP automated tissue processor or similar automated tissue processor. Briefly, the process involves the samples being dehydrated through ascending concentrations of ethanol, from 20% to 100% ethanol, cleared in xylene, and embedded in Paraplast Plus wax. Three-micron-thick sections for immunohistochemistry were cut and collected on SuperFrost Plus glass microscope slides.

3.3.2. Immunostaining of Tissue Sections

Tissue samples can be immunostained using a single primary antibody, or double-immunostained using two primary antibodies, as outlined in this section. It is not recommended that DAB be used as a chromogen, as the brown stain is not compatible with endogenous melanin in the skin.

There are a number of companies who supply kits for double immunostaining on paraffin-embedded tissue samples. A Histostain-DS kit for double immunostaining can be used to reveal two distinct antigens in a single tissue. Any combination of mouse, rabbit, rat, or guinea pig primary antibodies may be used. The Histostain-DS kits use the labeled streptavidin-biotin (LAB-SA) method, also known as streptavidin-biotin amplification. Two distinct substrate/chromogen/enzyme systems are used: BCIP/NBT/alkaline phosphatase, which produces a dark purple stain, and hydrogen peroxide/AEC/peroxidase, which produces an intense red stain. This kit has been designed to eliminate any interactions between the two staining systems. To enhance staining using established protocols, there is also a double stain enhancer, which is used after the first stain, and has been designed to enhance the second staining step.

Use of the double staining protocol allows the user to photograph the section after the first antigen has been visualized by mounting the section in water with a coverslip. This can be undertaken after the double stain enhancer has been incubated on the section. It is important that the time delay be kept to a minimum, and that water under the coverslip not evaporate, allowing the section to dry out. When using a double-immunostaining system, it is essential that one use a darker stain as the second stain; otherwise, it is difficult to examine co-localization of the two antigens. After the second antigen has been detected, the section can be permanently mounted and photographed.

3.3.3. Biochemical Analyses

The tissue samples can be homogenized for subsequent biochemical analyses. Protein or DNA can be readily extracted from the tissue sample.

1. Tissue is removed from the culturing medium, washed briefly in ice-cold PBS twice, and removed from the buffer. At this point the samples can be snap frozen and stored at $-70°C$.
2. Place the tissue in a petri dish, and use a scalpel to cut the tissue into small pieces.
3. Place the tissue immediately into ice-cold NETN buffer without the Nonidet P-40 (*see* **Note 8**) and homogenize using a polytron tissue homogenizer (Kinematica). Homogenize the tissue with ten 10-s bursts of the polytron, or until the sample is reduced to a mixture of even consistency. Throughout this procedure, maintain the sample on ice to minimize heating of the sample.
4. Add 1/20 volume of a 10% Nonidet P-40 solution and mix homogenate for 20 min with gentle agitation.
5. Centrifuge the sample at $1.35 \times 10^6 g$ in a Beckman TL-100 ultracentrifuge for 1 h at 4°C. Transfer the supernatant to a clean tube and store on ice.
6. Estimate the protein concentration of the samples using a BioRad DC protein assay. Aliquot the sample and store at $-70°C$.

The skin lysates can be used in the same manner as lysates prepared from cultured cells for a range of normal biochemical analyses, including fractionation, protein kinase assays, immunoprecipitation, Western blotting, and ELISAs.

7

Generation and Analysis of *Brca1* Conditional Knockout Mice

Chu-Xia Deng and Xiaoling Xu

Summary

Germline mutations of the breast tumor suppressor gene *BRCA1* predispose women to breast and ovarian cancers. However, loss-of-function mutations of mouse *Brca1* results in recessive embryonic lethality, which obscures the functions of *BRCA1* in breast cancer formation. Cre-loxP-mediated tissue-specific knockout was employed to overcome this obstacle. We found that the presence of a ploxP-*neo*-loxP cassette in intron 10 of *Brca1* resulted in severe interference with gene expression. The *neo* cassette was deleted in either embryonic stem cells or mice to generate the *neo*-less conditional knockout allele. Finally, we performed functional analysis of mammary tumorigenesis in *Brca1* conditional knockout mice. The methods to generate and analyze these *Brca1* conditional knockout mice are described in this chapter.

Key Words: Gene targeting; embryonic stem cell; mouse; MMTV-Cre; WAP-Cre; EIIa-Cre; LoxP; cell culture; chromosome spreads; mammary gland development; tumorigenesis.

1. Introduction

Breast cancer is the most common cancer and the second leading cause of cancer mortality in women (*1*). Germline mutations of *BRCA1* have been detected in approx 90% of combined familial breast and ovarian cancers, but in only approx 50% of familial breast cancers (*2–4*). Full-length BRCA1 is a nuclear protein of 220 kD containing 1863 amino acids in human and 1812 amino acids in mouse, respectively (*5,6*). The *BRCA1* gene encodes two major isoforms—the full-length isoform and the Δ-11 isoform, owing to alternative splicing at exon 11 (*7*). Exon 11 of *BRCA1* is the largest exon and encodes approx 60% of the protein. This exon contains two putative nuclear localiza-

From: *Methods in Molecular Biology, vol. 280: Checkpoint Controls and Cancer, Volume 1:*
Reviews and Model Systems
Edited by: Axel H. Schönthal © Humana Press Inc., Totowa, NJ

3. Methods

3.1. Generating the Conditional Targeting Vector for Brca1

An 18-kb fragment of genomic DNA containing the *Brca1* gene, which was isolated from a mouse genomic library derived from 129SVJ strain (Stratagene), is shown in **Fig. 2A**. The following four steps are used to insert the third loxP site into the *Eco*RI site in *Brca1* intron 11, and to prepare 3' arm for the *Brca1* conditional targeting vector.

1. Digest the plasmid (shown in **Fig. 2A**) with *Xho*I (arrows), followed by self-ligation. The resulting plasmid is shown in **Fig. 2B**. This step is necessary to make the *Cla*I site unique.
2. Digest the plasmid with *Cla*I (arrowheads), followed by self-ligation. The resulting plasmid is shown in **Fig. 2C**. This step is necessary to make the *Eco*RI site unique.
3. Digest the resulting plasmid with *Eco*RI (arrow, **Fig. 2C**) and fill the ends with Klenow polymerase to blunt the ends. Insert the oligos (**Fig. 1B**) containing the third loxP site. Digest the resulting construct with *Cla*I and *Not*I, and purify the fragment from agarose gel.
4. Digest the construct shown in **Fig. 2B** with *Cla*I and *Not*I; Insert the *Cla* I nd *Not* I fagment purified in **step 3**. The resulting construct (shown in **Fig. 2D**) contains a 5.5-kb fragment of the *Brca1* genomic DNA and a loxP site in intron 11.

The following three steps are used to prepare the 5' arm and ligate it to the *Brca1* targeting construct.

1. Digest the plasmid (shown in **Fig. 2A**) with *Eco*RV and *Xho*I (as indicated by asterisks), fill the ends with Klenow polymerase to blunt the ends, and purify the 3.5-kb *Eco*RV-*Xho*I fragment from agarose gel.
2. Digest the ploxPneo-1 plasmid (**Fig. 1A**) with *Xba*I and *Eco*RI, and blunt the ends with Klenow polymerase. Insert the *Eco*RV-*Xho*I fragment prepared in the previous step through blunt-end ligation (*see* **Note 1**). Screen clones for correct orientation using proper restriction enzymes (i.e. *Xba*I).
3. Digest the resulting construct with *Xho* I and *Not*I. Insert the 5.5-kb *Xho*I -*Not*I fragment containing the third loxP (**Fig. 2D**). The finished targeting construct, *ploxPneoBrca1*, is shown in **Fig. 2E** (*see* **Note 2**).

3.2. Generation of Brca1 Conditional Knockout ES Cells and Mice

The targeting vector (**Fig. 2E**) results in about 10% targeted ES clones (*10*). However, we found that the presence of the *neo* gene in intron 10 completely blocked normal splicing of the *Brca1* gene and caused embryonic lethality at around E8.5 (*15*). Therefore, we removed the *ploxPneo* gene using the following two approaches in ES cells and mouse germline, respectively.

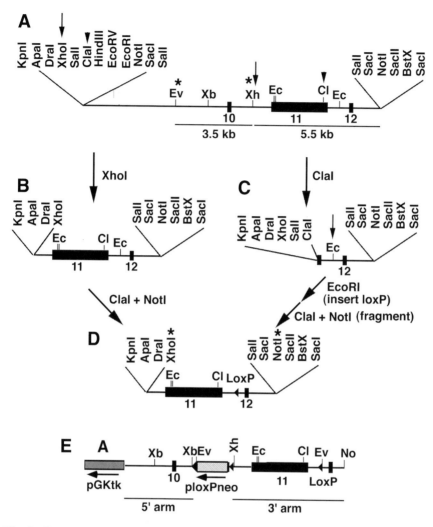

Fig. 2. Construction of the targeting vector for *Brca1*. (**A**) A 18-kb genomic fragment of the *Brca1* gene that has been cloned into the *Not*I site of pBluescript. This fragment was isolated from a 129SVJ-mouse genomic library (Stratagene). The *Sac*I and *Sal*I sites flanking the *Not*I sites are from phage arms. The 3.5 kb *Eco*RV-*Xho*I fragment, and the 5.5 kb *Xho*I-*Not*I fragment will be used as 5' and 3' arms of targeting vector respectively. (**B**) A 5.5-kb genomic fragment of *Brca1* generated by *Xho*I (arrows in **A**) digestion followed by recirculation (i.e., self-ligation) of the vector. (**C**) A 2.5 kb fragment of *Brca1* generated by *Cla*I (arrowheads in **A**) digestion followed by recirculation of the vector. (**D**) The 5.5-kb fragment of *Brca1* containing the third loxP site (triangle) in intron 11 of *Brca1*. (**E**) *Brca1* conditional targeting vector, *ploxPneoBrca1*. Ec, *Eco*RI; Ev, *Eco*RV; Xb, *Xba*I; Xh: *Xho*I. Numbered boxes are exons.

3.2.1. Removal of the ploxPneo From Targeted ES Cells

As shown in **Fig. 3A**, the *Brca1*floxed allele contains three loxP sites. Cre-mediated recombination could theoretically occur between any two of the three sites, generating offspring with three possible genotypes **(Fig. 3B)**. Mice with different genotypes can be identified by PCR analysis using four different primer pairs specifically designed for each Cre-mediated recombination event **(Fig. 3C)**. If recombination occurs between loxP sites 1 and 2, the *neo* gene is deleted, generating mice that contain loxP sites only in introns. Such an allele is likely to be true conditional knockout allele **(Fig. 3B-II)** .

In the original design, a negative marker, the thymidine kinase gene (tk), was used for selecting the Cre-mediated recombination that deleted the *neo* gene *(16)*. Because the targeted *Brca1* locus does not contain the *tk* gene, we performed the experiment with some modifications.

1. Grow ES cells that are heterozygous for the *ploxPneoBrca1* targeted allele (*Brca1neo-loxp/+*) (*see* **Note 3**).
2. Transfect 5 μg of the *pMC1-Cre* plasmid (unlinearized) into 10^7 ES cells using electroporation (25 μF, 600 mV, Bio-Rad gene pulser II).
3. Plate ES cells at densities of 500, 1000, 2000, and 3000 cells/10-cm plate, respectively. Change medium every day during the entire period of selection.
4. Seven days after electroporation, change the medium to PBS (10 mL). Draw three equally spaced parallel lines on the bottom of the plate containing the ES clones. Draw another three lines perpendicular to the previous lines.
5. Pick ES clones under an inverted microscope using a Pipetman P-200 with its volume adjusted to 20 μL and transfer the clones into a 96-well plate. A total of 384 clones (four 96-well plates) were picked for the *Brca1* project.
6. Add 50 μL of trypsin (diluted 1:1 with PBS) to each well and leave the plates at room temperature for 5 min. Add 100 μL of medium and pipet up and down 10× to disperse the cells. Duplicate the ES clones by transferring them (80 μL for each transfer) to two fresh 96-well plates. The first set of plates contains 100 μL of regular medium, and the second set of plates contains 100 μL of regular medium plus G418 at a concentration of 540 μg/mL. This is necessary to make the final concentration 300 μg/mL after the addition of the 80 μL solution containing ES cells.
7. Three days later, inspect both sets of plates under an inverted microscope and identify G418-sensitive clones by comparing the two sets of plates (G418-sensitive clones should be absent in the second set of plates and grow well in the first set of plates). Amplify the G418-sensitive clones from the first set of the plates by trypsinizing and transferring them to 24-well plates. Three days later, transfer to six-well plates.
8. After the ES cells have grown to cover most of the well, freeze two-thirds cells of each well in two vials. Prepare DNA from the remaining one-third cells for genotyping.

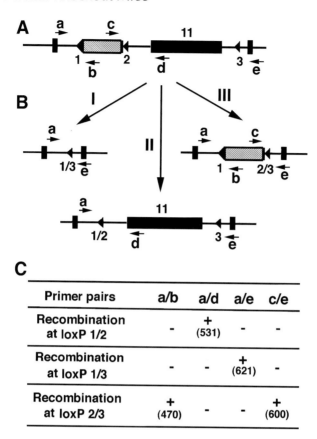

Fig. 3. *Brca1* conditional knockout allele and identification of Cre-mediated recombination. (**A**) Gene structure of the *Brca1*-floxed allele. Arrows represent PCR primers and their directions used in the assay. LoxP sites are indicated by numbers. (**B**) Three possible genotypes generated by Cre-mediated recombination. Genotypes II and III require partial excision between loxP 1 and 2 or loxP 2 and 3, while genotype I is a product from a complete deletion between loxP 1 and 3. (**C**) Primer pairs used for the detection of Cre-mediated recombination at all three possible sites. Numbers in parenthesis are the lengths of DNA fragments amplified by these primer pairs. The sequences for these primers are shown below:

a, 5'-CTGGGTAGTTTGTAAGCATGC-3',
b, 5'-GATATTGCTGAAGAGCTTGGC-3',
c, 5'-CCAGACTGCCTTGGGAAAAGC-3',
d, 5'-CAATAAACTGCTGGTCTCAGG-3',
e, 5'-CTGCGAGCAGTCTTCAGAAAG-3'.

Our data indicated that 44 out of 384 clones picked from transfected cells were G418 sensitive. Two out of 44 G418-sensitive clones contained recombination that removed just the *neo* gene. While this method has been used successfully in generating many strains (reviewed in *17*), it does require additional modification of ES cells and increases the difficulty of obtaining germline transmission. Moreover, the presence of *neo* in an intron of an endogenous gene can fortuitously create a hypomorphic allele, which may be useful in studying the function of genes of interest *(18–21)*. In such cases, it will be beneficial to remove the *neo* gene in the mouse after its effects are determined.

3.2.2. Excision of neo From Adult Mouse Using Ella-Cre Transgenic Mice

We next removed *neo* from the mouse germline by crossing the *Brca1neo-loxp/+* mice with a transgenic mouse carrying the *EIIa-Cre* transgene *(13)*. This is based on our previous finding that although the *EIIa-Cre* is quite potent for carrying out recombination in the mouse germline, it often yields partial recombination/excision between loxP sites *(22,23)*.

1. Cross female mice heterozygous for the floxed allele (*Brca1neo-loxp/+*) with *EIIa-Cre* homozygous male mice (**Fig. 4A**).
2. Analyze the tail DNA from 52 offspring by PCR to determine the recombination products present in each mouse (**Fig. 3C**). PCR analysis indicated that 30% of offspring carried a recombination between loxP sites 1 and 3, which deleted the entire region flanked by the loxP sites. Forty percent of the mice contained a mixture of *Brca1* alleles with recombination between loxP sites 1/2, 1/3, or 2/3, indicating that these mice were mosaics for partial and complete excisions.
3. Set up mating between mosaic F1 offspring to segregate the *Brca1* alleles generated by Cre-mediated recombination at the different loxP sites (**Fig. 4B**).
   For this experiment, we mated three pairs of mosaic F1 mice and found that 8 out of 43 (19%) F2 offspring had only the *neo* gene removed to produce a *neo*-less conditional knockout (recombination between loxP1 and loxP2, *Brca1loxp/+*). Three of these mice did not have the *EIIa-Cre* gene as a result of segregation. One normal *Brca1loxp/loxp* mouse was also generated, indicating that the deletion of *neo* rescued the embryonic lethal phenotype. *Brca1loxp/+* mice were also generated by crosses between wild-type mice and mosaic F1 mice (*see* **Note 4**).

3.3. Mammary Tissue-Specific Knockout of the Brca1 Gene

1. Cross *Brca1loxp/+* mice (to simplify the terminology, we have been calling this allele *Brca1Co/+* in our recent publications) with mice that carry either an *MMTV-Cre* or *WAP-Cre* transgene to generate *Brca1Co/CoMMTV-Cre* and *Brca1Co/CoWAP-Cre* mice (**Fig. 5A**). In our initial study, we also introduced a *Brca1*-null allele (*Brca1Ko*, ref *24*) to generate *Brca1Co/KoMMTV-Cre* and *Brca1Co/KoWAP-Cre* mice, so that one copy of *Brca1* is already deleted in these mice.
2. Monitor Cre-mediated recombination by PCR, or Northern and/or Southern blots. The *WAP-Cre* transgene is expressed almost exclusively in mammary tissue;

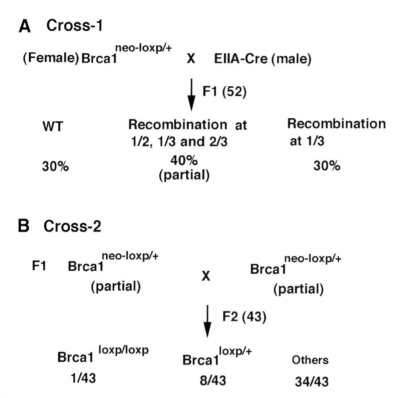

Fig. 4. Removal of the ploxP-neo-loxP from mouse germline by crossing with a transgenic mouse carrying *EIIa-Cre* gene. (**A**) Cross-1: Female mice heterozygous for the floxed allele (*BRCA1neo-loxp/+*) were crossed with male EIIa-Cre transgenic mice. The tail DNA from 52 offspring was analyzed by PCR using varying combinations of primers (*see* **Fig. 3C**). The PCR analysis indicated that 40% of the mice contained mixtures of recombination at loxP sites 1/2, 1/3, and 2/3, owing to partial excision by Cre recombinase. (**B**) Cross-2: Crossing of three pairs of mice containing the mixed recombination indicated that about 19% of offspring had the neo gene removed (recombination between LoxP 1 and 2, *Brca1loxp/+*), while leaving the third loxP site untouched. One *Brca1loxp/loxp* mouse was also generated by these crosses, indicating that deleting the *neo* gene rescued the embryonic lethal phenotype.

however, the *MMTV-Cre* transgene is active in many tissues. Northern blot analysis indicated that the *Brca1* transcripts were dramatically reduced in mammary tissue from P11.5 and P16.5 *Brca1Co/KoWAP-Cre* mice (**Fig. 5B**). Based on the intensities of the *Brca1* and GAPDH transcripts, the amount of transcripts from *Brca1Co/KoWAP-Cre* glands was less than 10% of control levels. This observation indicates that the Cre-loxP mediated approach disrupted *Brca1* in mammary epithelium with high efficiencies (*see* **Note 5**).

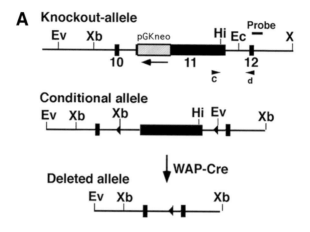

A **Knockout-allele**

Conditional allele

↓ **WAP-Cre**

Deleted allele

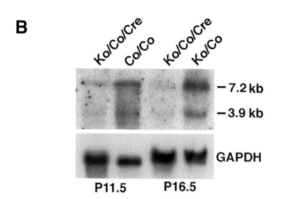

B

- 7.2 kb
- 3.9 kb

GAPDH

P11.5   P16.5

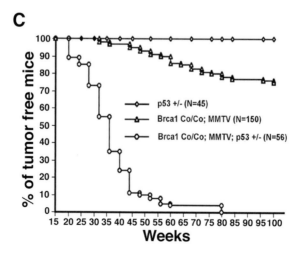

C

3.4. Monitor Mammary Gland Development by Whole-Mount Staining

1. Dissect out the fourth gland from each *Brca1* mutant mouse. Place it on a glass slides. Spread tissues using a forceps.
2. Fix the glands by dipping the slides into a 50-mL conical tube containing Caunoy's fixative for 1 h at room temperature (can be overnight).
3. Wash the glands with 70% ethanol for 15 min (can be stored after this wash for up to several months), followed by 50%, 30% ethanol and dH$_2$O for 5 min of each.
4. Stain with the carmine-aluminum stain at 4°C overnight.
5. Wash slides in ethanol baths of increasing concentrations (70-95-100%) for 15 min of each.
6. Transfer into xylene and mount them with Permount (Fisher).
7. Analyze the stained mammary glands under a dissecting microscope. Assess potential effects of the absence of *Brca1* on mammary gland development by comparing *Brca1* mutant glands with control glands prepared under identical conditions (*see* **Note 6**).

3.5. Tumorigenesis in Brca1 *Conditional Knockout Mice*

Brca1 conditional mutant mice started to develop mammary tumors at approx 10 mo of age, and by 1.5 yr of age, about 25% of the mice developed mammary tumors (**Fig. 5C**). We found that haploid loss of p53 significantly accelerated mammary tumorigenesis. In a studied population of 56 *Brca1Co/CoMMTV-CreP53+/-* mice, over half of the animals had mammary tumors by 8 mo of age, and all developed mammary tumors by 15 mo of age (**Fig. 5C**). Immunohistochemical staining detected extensive genetic/molecular alterations, including overexpression of ErbB2, c-Myc, p21, p27, and Cyclin D1, and downregulation of p16 (*25*). Further analysis revealed that a majority of tumors exhibited chromosomal abnormalities, with a pattern of chromosomal gain and loss that was similar to the pattern in human breast carcinomas (*26*).

Fig. 5. *(opposite page)* Targeted disruption of full-length isoform of *Brca1* in mammary gland results in tumor formation. (**A**) Genomic structure of the *Brca1* knockout allele (Ko) and the conditional allele (Co). (**B**) Northern blot analysis showing a sharp reduction of the *Brca1* transcripts in mammary glands isolated from P11.5 and P16.5 *Brca1Ko/Co;WAP-Cre* mice. A cDNA probe containing exons 10 and 12 of the *Brca1* gene was used for hybridization. Two major fragments of about 7.2 and 3.9 kb were detected in all samples. We have previously shown that the 3.9-kb transcript is a natural Δ11 product, which creates an in-frame fusion between exon 10 and exon 12, while the 7.2-kb band may represent the full-length transcripts (*7*). Note that both bands are much weaker in samples with the *WAP-Cre* transgene. The same filter was also hybridized with a GAPDH probe to provide a loading control. (**C**) Percentage of mice that are mammary tumor-free as a function of time for (1) *p53$^{+/-}$*; (2) *Brca1Co/Co;MMTV-Cre*; and (3) *Brca1Co/Co;MMTV-Cre;p53$^{+/-}$* genotypes.

3.6. Analysis of Brca1 *Mutant Tumors*

It is essential to establish cell lines from mammary tumors of mutant mice and perform phenotypic analysis at the cell-culture level. Here we describe the methods for mammary epithelial cell culture and chromosome spreads.

3.6.1. Derive Cell Lines From Mammary Tumors

1. Wash the tumor tissues with PBS twice. Mince them as small as possible with a sterile seizes] in a 10-cm plate. Add 10 MEGM media containing 10 µg/mL of bacterial collagenase type III. After overnight digestion at 37°C in a CO_2 culture incubator, pellet cells and finely minced tissues. Wash cells with PBS once and culture cells in MEGM media.
2. Monitor cultures for epithelial cell growth and change the medium every 3 d. When fibroblastic cells are depleted and only adherent epithelial cells remain (*see* **Note 7**), trypsinize the cultures and passage the cells. Once the cell lines are established, they can be maintained in DMEM supplemented with 5% FBS.

3.6.2. Chromosome Spreads

1. Plate 10^6 tumor cells into a 10-cm plate. Twenty-four hours later, treat the cells with colcemid for 1 h by directly adding the stock solution to culture medium at a final concentration of 0.01 µg/mL (10 mL/plate).
2. Remove the medium, trypsinize the cells, and transfer to a 10 mL conical centrifuge tube to pellet the cells.
3. Aspirate the medium and flick the tube to loosen the cell pellet. Resuspend the cells gently in 2 mL of 0.56% KCl and leave the tube at room temperature for 5 min.
4. Pre-fix the cells by adding 2 mL of ice-cold fixative (3:1 volumes of absolute methanol to glacial acetic acid, freshly prepared) along the side of the tube. Do not mix. Leave the tube at room temperature for 10 min.
5. Mix the cells by gently pipeting. Two minutes later, pellet the cells by gentle centrifugation (500 *g*, 2 min). Aspirate the supernatant and add 2 mL of fixative, followed by gently pipeting to suspend the cells in fixative. Leave the tube for 5 min at room temperature.
6. Change the fixative two more times by spinning out the cells. Then, suspend cells in 0.5 mL of fixative. The suspension can be used immediately to make chromosome spreads, or be stored at –20°C. In case of storage, change to freshly made ice-cold fixative before use.
7. For chromosome spreads, glass slides should be stored in –20°C with or without soaking in 70% alcohol. Use them quickly after taking out of the freezer.
8. Take a small quantity of fixed cells in a Pasteur pipet. Hold the pipet and position the end of it approx 20 cm above the slide. Release two or three drops of suspension at different positions of the slide. The drops spread quickly to reach the sides of the slides in a few seconds. A gentle blow across the surface of the slide can facilitate the spreading.

9. After air dry, the slides can be stained with Giemsa (based on manufacturer's instructions) or processed for spectral karyotyping *(10,27)*.
10. Analyze the spreads under the microscope (*see* **Note 8**).

4. Notes

1. Owing to the generally poor efficiency of blunt-end ligation, it might be difficult to insert the blunt-end fragment into *ploxPneo*. If this happens, the fragment can be inserted into pBluescript through its polylinker region to facilitate the screening by using blue/white selection. The fragment in pBluescript can be excised with proper restriction enzymes and cloned into *ploxPneo-1*.
2. In the *ploxPneo-1* vector, both *PGKneo* and *PGKtk* use about 500 bp for PGK-1 promoter and about 450 bp for PGK-1 terminator. These duplications sometimes generate instability during subcloning. To overcome this problem, we have generated *ploxPneo-2*, which uses *pMC1tk* to replace the *PGKtk*. The *pMC1tk* uses a *tk* promoter and a synthetic terminator to control *tk* gene expression *(28)*.
3. ES cells should be grown on mitomycin C-treated feeder cells made from mouse embryonic fibroblast cells. Culture medium needs to be changed every day for growing ES cells.
4. We have described two approaches to delete the *neo* gene. At least three other approaches have been reported. The first uses a combination of Cre/loxP and FLP/FRT systems. The *neo* gene is flanked by two FRT sites, so that the deletion of the *neo* gene by FLP recombinase does not affect the loxP-flanked fragment *(29)*. The second and third approaches inject Cre directly into oocytes and blastocysts, respectively *(16,30)*. They all reportedly work successfully in deleting the *neo* gene.
5. The *MMTV-Cre* transgene is active in many tissues *(31)*. Although it does not cause an obvious abnormality in other tissues in *Brca1Co/CoMMTV-Cre* mice, it does cause skin abnormalities in some other conditional knockout mice (i.e., *Smad4Co/CoMMTV-Cre* mice; our unpublished observation). Therefore, *WAP-Cre* should be a better choice if the floxed gene of interest is known to have essential functions in other tissues/organs.
6. Morphology of mammary glands is different at each phase during mammary cycle of development. The minimum time points that need to be examined include virgin mice of 3, 4, 5, and 6 wk, pregnancy d 12 and 16, lactation d 1 and 10, involution d 2 and 10. Pay close attention to branch morphogenesis, alveolar densities, and mammary tree structures. Suspected abnormal areas should be further examined by histological sections.
7. Depletion of fibroblastic cells requires invariably long time (e.g., 1–6 mo). Because epithelial cells attach to the culture dish much better than fibroblasts, the gentle treatment of cells with diluted trypsin (1:1 with PBS) for 2–5 min, followed by a PBS wash, can help to remove fibroblasts. This procedure may be repeated a few times on different days, until a pure population of epithelial cells is obtained.

5. Chromosomal abnormalities can also be noted during the scan for mitotic cells. Analyze each mitotic chromosome spread and score for abnormalities (aneuploidy, chromosome breaks, chromosome fusions). Spectral karyotyping methods can be applied to distinguish different chromosomes and detect translocations *(12)*.

3.2.5. Cell Cycle and Checkpoint Analysis

Because M-phase accumulation in the presence of nocodazole represents progression of interphase cells through S/G2, a limited analysis of checkpoint function may also be possible with the procedures described in **Subheadings 3.2.2.** through **3.2.4.**. Checkpoint functions can be determined by treating blastocysts with DNA-damaging agents or DNA-replication inhibitors and then adding nocodazole to measure the percentage of cells capable of overriding checkpoint controls and entering mitosis. Of course, all of the caveats for the procedure described in **Subheading 3.2.2.** should also be applied to any assessment of checkpoint function.

3.3. PCR Genotyping Early Embryonic Cultures

The methods described in **Subheadings 3.1.** and **3.2.** require genotype identification by PCR. Although genotyping can be problematic given how little DNA can be isolated, Southern blotting the PCR products to nylon membrane and probing with a radiolabeled primer specific to internal regions of the amplified DNA can enhance the signal of the amplified DNA and decrease the nonspecific signal derived from background amplification events. The internal primer probe should recognize both the wild-type and mutant PCR products but should not overlap with any of the primers used for amplification.

3.3.1. DNA Preparation

1. Wash cells from **Subheading 3.1.3.** or **3.2.3., step 4**, three times in PBS (*see* **Note 8**). Be sure to use aerosol-resistant tips for all pipeting. For experiments using cells from **Subheading 3.1.3.**, use the washing procedures described in **Subheading 3.2.3., step 1**. For experiments using cells from **Subheading 3.2.3., step 4**, follow the washing procedure described in **Subheading 3.2.3., steps 5** and **6**.
2. Carefully remove all but approx 2 µL of the PBS supernatant with a P20 pipet aid.
3. Add 2 µL of 2X NSPK buffer and vortex gently.
4. To prepare DNA from cells described in **Subheading 3.1.3.**, wrap plates in parafilm, cover with the lid, and incubate at 37°C for 20 min to lyse/detach cells; following the incubation, pipet the entire 4 µL into a 200 µL PCR tube. To prepare DNA from cells described in **Subheading 3.2.3., step 4**, proceed to **step 5** below.

5. Cap tubes and incubate for 4 h at 60°C, followed by a 30 min incubation at 90°C to inactivate the proteinase K (*see* **Note 9**).
6. Freeze DNA at -20°C or proceed to **Subheading 3.3.2.**.

3.3.2. PCR, Southern Blotting, and Oligonucleotide Probing

1. Add primers and PCR mix to the entire DNA preparation from **Subheading 3.3.1.** above and run a 25 µL PCR. PCR reactions can and should be run in the same tubes in which the DNA was prepared (*see* **Note 8**). For any given mutant, the PCR conditions previously developed for tail DNA genotyping of the knockout in question should be used.
2. Separate PCR reaction products on a TBE/agarose gel containing ethidium bromide.
3. Photograph gel to document ethidium bromide-stained molecular-weight standards.
4. Incubate gel for 30 min in denaturing solution and Southern blot onto nylon membrane (Hybond N+) by capillary transfer overnight in denaturing solution.
5. Bake the membrane for 2 h at 80°C in a vacuum oven.
6. End-label 60 pmol of a single-stranded oligonucleotide (24–30 bp) that is specific for an internal region of the PCR product (i.e., does not overlap with amplification primer sequence) by incubating it with 20 U T4 PNK, 1X reaction buffer, and 150 µCi ^{32}P-γ-ATP for 30 min at 37°C. Remove unincorporated ^{32}P-γ-ATP by G-25 column chromatography.
7. Hybridize the filter with $0.5–1 \times 10^6$ cpm/mL oligonucleotide probe in SSDS for 3 h at a temperature that is 40°C below the calculated Tm for oligonucleotide annealing to the PCR products.
8. Wash the filter five times for 15 min each in 1X SSPE/0.1% SDS at the same temperature used for hybridization.
9. Wrap filter in plastic wrap and expose the hybridized membrane to film or PhosphorImager (Molecular Dynamics) to identify blastocyst genotypes.

3.4. Complementation Through Lentiviral Transgenesis?

Complemention of one-cell zygotes with the Cre/lox-conditional form of the disrupted gene's cDNA could theoretically prevent ICM loss during subsequent culture of mutant blastocysts. While conventional transgenesis techniques such as pronuclear injections could be used for such a procedure, the efficiency of pronuclear injection is low and often results in multiple integrants that would make Cre/lox-mediated deletion problematic. A method that overcomes both of these obstacles has recently been developed (*9*). This method uses lentiviruses to efficiently transduce one-cell zygotes in culture. Besides its high efficiency, lentiviral transgenesis offers a particular advantage over pronuclear injections in that single-copy integrants are possible. This provides an opportunity to complement knockout zygotes with a Cre/lox-conditional form of the disrupted gene. Once cell lines have been established from cultured blastocysts, this floxed transgene could then be conditionally deleted by intro-

We have designed two techniques that monitor the formation of DSBs, and we have used them successfully to demonstrate that DSBs arise during DNA replication in the absence of X-Mre11. The first technique is based on the direct labeling of DNA containing DSBs by terminal transferase, whereas the second technique uses indirect labeling of chromatin protein using an antibody against phosphorylated histone H2AX. Terminal transferase covalently adds dNTP to 3'-OH of deoxynucleotides. H2AX is a histone variant that specifically becomes phosphorylated in presence of DSBs. Phospho-H2AX is detected in nucleosomes that are in proximity to the breaks *(29,30)*. Details of these protocols follow.

3.5.2.1. TUNEL Assay

1. Incubate 50 µL of control interphase extract (*see* **Subheading 3.1.2.**) or extract in which the occurrence of DSBs will be assessed, with 10,000 nuclei/µL for 120 min at 20°C.
2. Dilute extracts in 1 mL of a buffer consisting of 100 mM KCl, 25 mM HEPES (pH 7.8), 2.5 MgCl$_2$, and 0.4% Triton X-100.
3. Layer samples onto the same buffer containing 30% sucrose without Triton and spin for 20 min at 6000g in a HB-6 rotor (Sorvall).
4. Wash pellets and incubate at 37°C for 4 h in a buffer containing 90 U of terminal transferase, 100 mM potassium cacodylate (pH 7.0), 1 mM CoCl$_2$, 0.2 mM DTT, 25 µCi dGTP, 3,000 Ci/mM, and 50 µM dGTP.
5. Incubate control reactions in the same buffer without TdT.
6. Treat reaction mixtures with 0.1 mg/mL proteinase K and extract the DNA with phenol-chloroform, then electrophorese on a 0.5% agarose gel at 100 V for 60 min.
7. Fix the gel in 20% TCA, dry, and expose for autoradiography.
8. Excise the labeled band from the gel and quantify by scintillation counting (*see* **Note 9**).

3.5.2.2. Phosphorylated Histone H2AX Detection

1. Incubate 50 µL of control interphase extract (*see* **Subheading 3.1.2.**) or extract in which the occurrence of DSBs will be assessed, with 10,000 nuclei/µL for 90 min at 23°C.
2. Isolate postreplicative chromatin by diluting the extracts in chromatin isolation buffer containing 1 mM NaF, 1 mM sodium vanadate, and 0.125% Triton X-100.
3. Layer samples onto chromatin isolation buffer containing 30% sucrose and lacking Triton X-100, then spin at 6000g for 20 min at 4°C.
4. Prepare a positive control by incubating sperm nuclei for 30 min in interphase extract to decondense chromatin.
5. Isolate the chromatin and digest for 4 h with *Not*I.

6. Reisolate the digested chromatin through a sucrose cushion and incubate in interphase extract for 60 min.
7. Boil chromatin in Laemmli buffer and process for sodium dodecyl sulfate-polyacrylamide gel electrophoresis (SDS-PAGE).
8. Use antiphosphorylated H2AX antibody for Western blotting at 1/6000 dilution.

4. Notes

1. The homogeneity of cytosolic extracts is critical to the success of all procedures; therefore, extracts need to be mixed several times by pipetting very gently but very thoroughly, to avoid formation of aggregates.
2. Depending on age and size, a female *Xenopus* will lay between 5 and 10 mL of dejellied eggs. This yields between 2 and 4 mL of egg cytosol.
3. The cytoplasmic layer can be pipetted by directly sliding a pipet tip against the wall of the tube through the top lipid layer. Alternatively, the lipid layer can be removed first using a cotton swab.
4. Cytosolic extracts (CSF or activated) must be used immediately after preparation. Freezing and thawing the extract triggers apoptosis.
5. For M/B fractionation, the quality of the eggs and the timing of the preparation is critical to get functional fractions. We perform the fractionation as soon as possible following the preparation of the extract. The complete procedure should not take more than 3 h to recover functional fractions. The quality of M and B fractions can also be tested in pilot experiments. M or B fractions do not support DNA replication by themselves, but only in combination. If background replication is observed with either M or B fraction alone, the concentration of PEG used for fractionation can be modified with a 1% window: $3.5 \pm 0.5\%$ for B and $9 \pm 0.5\%$ for M.
6. The stability of damaged DNA templates can be evaluated following incubation in cell-free extracts. 5' DNA termini and 3' DNA termini are labeled with T4 kinase and TdT, respectively (Gibco labeling kits).
7. The GST-peptide fusion protein described in **Subheading 3.3.** can be modified and replaced by any SQ-containing peptide known to be phosphorylated following DNA damage.
8. Some antigens tested for chromatin binding can be very abundant in the cytosolic fraction, as well as in the chromatin-bound fraction. It is therefore critical to avoid cytoplasmic contamination during the chromatin isolation step. To reduce background owing to cytoplasmic contamination of chromatin pellets, we further centrifuge interphase extract for 30 min at $13,000g$ at 4 °C. Furthermore, the chromatin pellets are isolated after freezing the bottom of the Eppendorf tube in liquid nitrogen by cutting the tip of the tube with scissors. We recover the pellet from the tip of the tube, resuspending it in Laemmli buffer.
9. For TUNEL assay, it is critical to check whether the extract has supported DNA replication. An aliquot of replicating extract can be incubated with α-^{32}P-dATP, processed, and run on the gel to monitor the DNA replication.

Acknowledgments

This work was supported by grants from the ACS (RSG CCG-103367) and the NCI (RO1 CA95866, RO1 CA92245) to J. G.

References

1. Hensey, C. and Gautier, J. (1995) Regulation of cell cycle progression following DNA damage. *Prog. Cell Cycle Res.* **1,** 149–162.
2. Zhou, B. B. and Elledge, S. J. (2000) The DNA damage response: putting checkpoints in perspective. *Nature* **408,** 433–439.
3. Murray, A. W. (1995) The genetics of cell cycle checkpoints. *Curr. Opin. Genet. Dev.* **5,** 5–11.
4. Beamish, H., Williams, R., Chen, P., and Lavin, M. F. (1996) Defect in multiple cell cycle checkpoints in ataxia-telangiectasia postirradiation. *J. Biol. Chem.* **271,** 20,486–20,493.
5. Petrini, J. H. (2000) The Mre11 complex and ATM: collaborating to navigate S phase. *Curr. Opin. Cell Biol.* **12,** 293–296.
6. Shiloh, Y. (1997) Ataxia-telangiectasia and the Nijmegen breakage syndrome: related disorders but genes apart. *Annu. Rev. Genet.* **31,** 635–662.
7. Blow, J. J. and Laskey, R. A. (1986) Initiation of DNA replication in nuclei and purified DNA by a cell-free extract of *Xenopus* eggs. *Cell* **47,** 577–587.
8. Gautier, J., Minshull, J., Lohka, M., Glotzer, M., Hunt, T., and Maller, J. L. (1990) Cyclin is a component of maturation-promoting factor from *Xenopus*. *Cell* **60,** 487–494.
9. Gautier, J., Norbury, C., Lohka, M., Nurse, P., and Maller, J. (1988) Purified maturation-promoting factor contains the product of a *Xenopus* homolog of the fission yeast cell cycle control gene *cdc2+*. *Cell* **54,** 433–439.
10. Gautier, J., Solomon, M. J., Booher, R. N., Bazan, J. F., and Kirschner, M. W. (1991) Cdc25 is a specific tyrosine phosphatase that directly activates p34cdc2. *Cell* **67,** 197–211.
11. Lohka, M. J. and Masui, Y. (1983) Formation in vitro of sperm pronuclei and mitotic chromosomes induced by amphibian ooplasmic components. *Science* **220,** 719–721.
12. Murray, A. W. and Kirschner, M. W. (1989) Cyclin synthesis drives the early embryonic cell cycle. *Nature* **339,** 275–280.
13. Murray, A. W., Solomon, M. J., and Kirschner, M. W. (1989) The role of cyclin synthesis and degradation in the control of maturation promoting factor activity. *Nature* **339,** 280–286.
14. Guo, Z. and Dunphy, W. G. (2000) Response of *Xenopus* Cds1 in cell-free extracts to DNA templates with double-stranded ends. *Mol. Biol. Cell.* **11,** 1535–1546.
15. Guo, Z., Kumagai, A., Wang, S. X., and Dunphy, W. G. (2000) Requirement for Atr in phosphorylation of Chk1 and cell cycle regulation in response to DNA replication blocks and UV-damaged DNA in *Xenopus* egg extracts. *Genes Dev.* **14,** 2745–2756.

16. Kumagai, A., Guo, Z., Emami, K. H., Wang, S. X., and Dunphy, W. G. (1998) The *Xenopus* Chk1 protein kinase mediates a caffeine-sensitive pathway of checkpoint control in cell-free extracts. *J. Cell Biol.* **142,** 1559–1569.

17. Kumagai, A., Yakowec, P. S., and Dunphy, W. G. (1998) 14-3-3 proteins act as negative regulators of the mitotic inducer Cdc25 in *Xenopus* egg extracts. *Mol. Biol. Cell.* **9,** 345–354.

18. Costanzo, V., Robertson, K., Ying, C. Y., et al. (2000) Reconstitution of an ATM-dependent checkpoint that inhibits chromosomal DNA replication following DNA damage. *Mol. Cell.* **6,** 649–659.

19. Costanzo, V., Shechter, D., Lupardus, P., et al. (2003) An ATR- and Cdc7-dependent DNA damage checkpoint that inhibits initiation of DNA replication. *Mol. Cell.* **11,** 203–213.

20. Costanzo, V., Robertson, K., Bibikova, M., et al. (2001) Mre11 protein complex prevents double-strand break accumulation during chromosomal DNA replication. *Mol. Cell.* **8,** 137–147.

21. Murray, A. W. (1991) Cell cycle extracts. *Methods Cell Biol.* **36,** 581–605.

22. Chong, J. P., Mahbubani, H. M., Khoo, C. Y., and Blow, J. J. (1995) Purification of an MCM-containing complex as a component of the DNA replication licensing system. *Nature* **375,** 418–421.

23. Chong, J. P., Thommes, P., Rowles, A., Mahbubani, H. M., and Blow, J. J. (1997) Characterization of the *Xenopus* replication licensing system. *Methods Enzymol.* **283,** 549–564.

24. Khanna, K. K., Lavin, M. F., Jackson, S. P., and Mulhern, T. D. (2001) ATM, a central controller of cellular responses to DNA damage. *Cell Death Differ.* **8,** 1052–1065.

25. Kim, S.T., Lim, D. S, Canman, C. E., and Kastan, M. B. (1999) Substrate specificities and identification of putative substrates of ATM kinase family members. *J. Biol. Chem.* **274,** 37,538–37,543.

26. Burden, D. A. and Osheroff, N. (1998) Mechanism of action of eukaryotic topoisomerase II and drugs targeted to the enzyme. *Biochim. Biophys. Acta* **1400,** 139–154.

27. Sarkaria, J. N., Busby, E. C., Tibbetts, R. S., et al. (1999) Inhibition of ATM and ATR kinase activities by the radiosensitizing agent, caffeine. *Cancer Res.* **59,** 4375–4382.

28. Robertson, K., Hensey, C., and Gautier, J. (1999) Isolation and characterization of *Xenopus* ATM (X-ATM): expression, localization, and complex formation during oogenesis and early development. *Oncogene* **18,** 7070–7079.

29. Rogakou, E. P., Boon, C., Redon, C., and Bonner, W. M. (1999) Megabase chromatin domains involved in DNA double-strand breaks in vivo. *J. Cell Biol.* **146,** 905–916.

30. Rogakou, E. P., Pilch, D. R., Orr, A. H., Ivanova, V. S., and Bonner, W. M. (1998) DNA double-stranded breaks induce histone H2AX phosphorylation on serine 139. *J. Biol. Chem.* **273,** 5858–5868.

10

A *Xenopus* Cell-Free System for Analysis of the Chfr Ubiquitin Ligase Involved in Control of Mitotic Entry

Dongmin Kang, Jim Wong, and Guowei Fang

Summary

The checkpoint protein Chfr delays entry into mitosis in the presence of mitotic stress. We have analyzed the Chfr checkpoint pathway in the *Xenopus* cell-free system. We showed that Chfr is a ubiquitin ligase that targets polo-like kinase (Plk1) for degradation, leading to delayed activation of the Cdc25C phosphatase and prolonged inhibitory phosphorylation of Cdc2 at the G2/M transition. In this chapter, we will describe biochemical methods we developed to analyze the Chfr auto-ubiquitination activity and the ubiquitination of its substrate Plk1, as well as functional assays to investigate the Chfr pathway in *Xenopus* extracts.

Key Words: Chfr; Plk1; Cdc2; Cdc25C; Wee1; cyclin B; mitotic entry; ubiquitin ligase; proteolysis; *Xenopus* cycling extracts.

1. Introduction

Entry into mitosis is controlled by a checkpoint pathway involving the ubiquitin ligase Chfr (*1,2*). In normal human cell lines, this checkpoint pathway functions at the G2 to M transition to delay condensation of chromosomes in response to drugs, such as Taxol and nocodazole, that disrupt microtubule structure (*3*). A key component of the checkpoint is the Chfr (checkpoint with FHA and ring finger) protein, which delays chromosome condensation and nuclear envelope breakdown in response to mitotic stress induced by Taxol or nocodazole. In several human tumor cell lines examined, the Chfr gene is either mutated or not expressed, and the Chfr checkpoint does not function. Ectopic expression of Chfr in these cells restores the cell cycle delay, indicating that Chfr is required for the checkpoint control (*1*). Expression of Chfr is also abolished in several types of primary tumors as a result of methylation of the gene promoter, suggesting that inhibition of Chfr expression provides proliferative advantage to tumor cells (*4–6*).

From: *Methods in Molecular Biology, vol. 280: Checkpoint Controls and Cancer, Volume 1: Reviews and Model Systems*
Edited by: Axel H. Schön thal © Humana Press Inc., Totowa, NJ

The Chfr protein contains three separate domains: an N-terminal forkhead-associated (FHA) domain, a central ring finger (RF) domain, and a C-terminal cysteine-rich (CR) domain. Based on mutagenesis analysis, both the FHA and CR domains are required for the checkpoint function (*1*). We found that Chfr is a ubiquitin ligase, and that the RF domain is both necessary and sufficient for its auto-ubiquitination activity (*2*). We have developed a cell-free system to analyze the biological function of the Chfr ligase. When added to *Xenopus* extracts, recombinant Chfr delays the activation of the Cdc2 kinase during the G2 to M transition, and this delay is caused by a prolonged inhibitory phosphorylation of tyrosine 15 on Cdc2. The target of the Chfr ligase is the polo-like kinase 1 (Plk1), and ubiquitination and degradation of Plk1 delays mitotic entry. Thus, Chfr represents a novel ubiquitin ligase involved in cell cycle regulation, and our biochemical analysis of Chfr function in *Xenopus* extracts provides a molecular mechanism for Chfr-mediated checkpoint control at the G2 to M transition (*2*). In this chapter, we will describe detailed methods for (1) expression and purification of the Chfr protein and other ubiquitination enzymes required for analysis of the Chfr ubiquitin ligase activity; (2) preparation of *Xenopus* cell cycle extracts; and (3) analysis of Chfr function in *Xenopus* extracts.

2. Materials

2.1. Expression and Purification of Recombinant Proteins

1. Bac-to-Bac Baculovirus Expression System and *Sf9* cells (Gibco).
2. BL21, BL21(DE3), and BL21(DE3)pLys cells (Novagen).
3. Ni-NTA agarose (Qiagen).
4. Glutathione agarose (Pharmacia).
5. Resource Q column (Pharmacia).
6. Ubiquitin-Affigel (BioRad).
7. Phenylmethylsulfonyl fluoride (PMSF) (Sigma).
8. Creatine phosphate (Sigma).
9. Phosphocreatine kinase (Sigma).
10. Chfr lysis buffer: 20 mM Tris-HCl, pH 8.5, 100 mM KCl, 1% NP-40, 2 mM PMSF, plus leupeptin, chymostatin, and pepstin, each at 10μg/mL.
11. Chfr/Ubc4 dialysis buffer: 10 mM Tris-HCl, pH 7.7, 100 mM KCl, and 1 mM DTT.
12. E1 lysis buffer: 50 mM Tris-HCl, pH 8.0, 1 mM EDTA, 0.2 mM DTT.
13. E1 wash buffer: 50 mM Tris-HCl, pH 8.0, and 500 mM KCl.
14. E1 elution buffer: 50 mM Tris-HCl, pH 9.0, and 10 mM DTT.
15. E1 dialysis buffer: 50 mM Tris-HCl, pH 7.5, and 1 mM DTT.
16. Thioester reaction buffer: 5 mM Tris-HCl, pH 7.7, 10 mM MgCl$_2$, 1 mM ATP, and 0.1 mM DTT. Store at 4°C.

17. Thioester sample buffer: 120 mM Tris-HCl, pH 6.8, 4% SDS, 4 M urea, and 20% glycerol. Store at 4°C.
18. Δ90CycB lysis buffer: 10 mM Tris-HCl, pH 8.0, 50 mM NaCl, 1 mM EDTA, 5 mM DTT, 0.05% NP40, and 2 mM PMSF. Store at 4°C.
19. Δ90CycB refolding buffer: 50 mM Tris-HCl, pH 8.0, 100 mM KCl, 5 mM MgCl$_2$, and 5 mM DTT. Store at 4°C.
20. QuikChange® Site-Directed Mutagenesis Kit (Stratagene).
21. Slide-A-Lyzer® (Pierce).
22. CentriPrep-10 (Pharmacia).

2.2. Preparation of Xenopus Extracts

1. Ca^{2+} Ionophore (A23187) (Calbiochem).
2. Human chorionic gonadotropin (hCG) (Sigma).
3. Pregnant mare serum gonadotropin (PMSG) (Calbiochem).
4. Cytochalasin B (1000X = 10 mg/mL) (Sigma).
5. Cycloheximide (100X = 10 mg/mL) (Sigma).
6. Protease inhibitor mix (leupeptin, chymostatin, and pepsin; 1000X = 10 mg/mL each) (Sigma).
7. Nyosil-M25 oil (ANDPAK-EMA).
8. MMR buffer: 100 mM NaCl, 2 mM KCl, 2 mM CaCl$_2$, 1 mM MgCl$_2$, 0.1 mM EDTA, and 5 mM HEPES, pH 7.7.
9. XB buffer: 10 mM HEPES, pH 7.7, 100 mM KCl, 0.1 mM CaCl$_2$, 1 mM MgCl$_2$, and 50 mM sucrose.
10. Energy regenerating system: 150 mM creatine phosphate, 20 mM ATP, pH 7.4, and 20 mM MgCl$_2$.

2.3. Analysis of the Chfr Ubiquitin Ligase

1. HEK293T cells (ATCC).
2. [^{35}S]-methionine (Pharmacia).
3. [^{32}P]-γ-ATP (Pharmacia).
4. [^{125}I]-Ubiquitin (NEN).
5. Ubiquitin (Ub) (Sigma)
6. Histone H1 (Calbiochem).
7. Chloramine T (Sigma).
8. Mouse anti-Myc antibody (9E10 clone) (Santa Cruz Biotechnology, Inc.).
9. HEK293T lysis buffer: 50 mM Tris-HCl, pH 7.7, 150 mM NaCl, 0.5% NP-40, 1 mM DTT, 10% glycerol, 0.5 μM okadaic acid, and 10 μg/mL each of leupeptin, pepstatin, and chymostatin.
10. EB buffer: 80 mM β-glycerophosphate, pH 7.4, 15 mM MgCl$_2$, 10 mM EGTA, and 0.1% NP-40.
11. TNT Coupled Transcription/Translation System (Promega).
12. PhosphorImager (Molecular Dynamics).

3. Methods

3.1. Expressing and Purifying Recombinant Proteins

3.1.1. Expressing and Purifying the Chfr Ligase From Sf9 Cells

1. Clone human Chfr gene by PCR amplification into the pFastBac vector.
2. Package the Chfr gene in the pFastBac vector into baculovirus following manufacturer's instructions.
3. Express the Chfr ligase in insect *Sf9* cells as a His-tagged recombinant protein (*see* **Note 1**). Infect 6 L of *Sf9* cells at a MOI of 5 with the Chfr baculovirus, and harvest cells 72 h postinfection. His-Chfr protein expressed in *Sf9* cells is soluble.
4. Lyse *Sf9* cells on ice in 5 vol of Chfr lysis buffer. Incubate lysates on ice for 30 min, sonicate for 2 min at 80% of maximal power output, and centrifuge at 20,000g for 30 min at 4°C.
5. Fractionate cleared supernatants over a 45-mL Resource Q anion exchange column (Pharmacia) at a flow rate of 5 mL/min. Elute bound proteins with a 300-mL linear salt gradient of 100 mM to 600 mM KCl and collect 14-mL fractions. Identify the peak of the Chfr protein by SDS-PAGE electrophoresis.
6. Purify the recombinant Chfr protein in peak fractions by Ni-NTA beads (**Fig. 1A**).
7. Dialyze the purified protein against the Chfr dialysis buffer, aliquot, and store at −80°C. The yield of purification is usually 1 mg Chfr protein per L of *Sf9* cells. The purified Chfr protein is stable for over 3 yr at −80°C.

To analyze the minimal domain of Chfr sufficient for its auto-ubiquitination, three deletion mutants were constructed by PCR subcloning. ChfrF1 (aa 1–360) contains both the FHA domain and the RF domain. ChfrF2 (aa 142–360) contains the RF domain and the spacer between the FHA and RF domains. GST–ChfrF3 (aa 267–360) has the RF domain fused to GST at its N-terminus (*see* **Note 2**). These recombinant proteins were expressed in BL21(DE3) (for ChfrF1 and 2) or in BL21 (for GST–ChfrF3). His–ChfrF1 and His–ChfrF2 were purified by Ni-NTA beads and GST–ChfrF3 was purified by glutathione-agarose beads.

To analyze the requirement of the ring-finger domain for Chfr ligase activity, two variants, ChfrI306A and ChfrW332A, with mutations in the conserved residues in the ring-finger domain, were constructed by QuikChange® Site-Directed Mutagenesis Kit. Mutant proteins were expressed and purified similarly to the wild-type protein.

3.1.2. Expressing and Purifying the Ubiquitin-Activating Enzyme

Ubiquitin-activating enzyme (E1) was purified through a ubiquitin-affinity column by the formation of the E1-ubiquitin thioester conjugate (*see* **Note 3**).

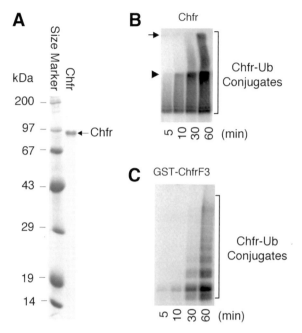

Fig. 1. Auto-ubiquitination of Chfr. (**A**) Purified recombinant Chfr protein assayed by 12% SDS-PAGE. Recombinant Chfr (**B**) and GST–ChfrF3 (**C**) were incubated with radioactive ubiquitin in the presence of E1 and Ubc4. The kinetics of the formation of the Chfr–ub conjugates was assayed by 12% reducing SDS-PAGE. The arrow points to the wells of the stacking gel and the arrowhead indicates the junction between stacking and separating gels.

1. Clone the E1 gene into a pET vector and express the E1 protein in 6 L of BL21(DE3). Spin down cell pellets.
2. Resuspend pellets from each liter of cells in 20 mL of E1 lysis buffer and lyse cells by sonication for 2 min at 80% of maximal power output. Immediately after sonication, add PMSF to 2 mM and MgCl$_2$ to 5 mM.
3. Centrifuge cell lysates at 12,000g for 30 min and then add ATP, creatine phosphate, and phosphocreatine kinase to supernatants at 2mM, 10 mM, and 5 U/mL, respectively.
4. Incubate cleared cell lysates with 3 mL of Ubiquitin-Affigel (6 mg ubiquitin/mL beads) for 2 h at room temperature, with gentle mixing at 30 rotations per min. Wash the ubiquitin column with 5 column vols of E1 wash buffer and elute the E1 protein with 3 vols of E1 elution buffer at a rate of 1 mL/min.
5. Concentrate eluted E1 by CentriPrep-10 and dialyze in a Slide-A-Lyzer against the E1 dialysis buffer. Aliquot the E1 protein and store at –80°C. The expected yield is about 0.5 mg E1 per L of *E. coli* culture.

3.1.3. Expressing and Purifying the Ubiquitin-Conjugating Enzyme (Ubc4)

1. Clone human Ubc4 into the pET28a vector by PCR amplification from human fetal thymus cDNA.
2. Express recombinant proteins in BL21(DE3) and purify by Ni-NTA beads. Identify the peak of the Ubc4 fractions by SDS-PAGE electrophoresis.
3. Further purify the peak of Ubc4 fractions over a 1-mL HiTrap Q column and dialyze purified protein against the Ubc4 dialysis buffer.

The activity of Ubc4 was assayed in a thioester assay.

1. Incubate the Ubc4 protein at room temperature for 5 min with 30 µg/mL labeled ubiquitin, 200 µg/mL recombinant E1, and 1 mM ATP. Perform the reaction in a total vol of 10 µL in the thioester reaction buffer with the final concentration of Ubc4 at 20 µg/mL.
2. Stop the reaction by addition of 10 µL of thioester sample buffer.
3. Analyze the reaction product by nonreducing 15% SDS-PAGE.

3.1.4. Expressing and Purifying the Nondegradable Cyclin B

Deletion of the N-terminal 90 amino acids from *Xenopus* cyclin B1 prevents its degradation by the anaphase-promoting complex pathway during mitosis *(7)*. This non-degradable form, Δ90CycB, stably arrests *Xenopus* extracts at mitosis upon its addition to interphase extracts.

1. Express the Δ90CycB protein in BL21(DE3)pLys as inclusion bodies *(7)*.
2. Resuspend the pellet from 1 L of cells in 25 mL of Δ90CycB lysis buffer. Lyse cells by sonication for 2 min.
3. Centrifuge cell lysates at 17,000g for 15 min. Wash cell pellets/inclusion bodies in the Δ90CycB lysis buffer plus 500 mM NaCl. Centrifuge again.
4. Resuspend cell pellets/inclusion bodies in 15 mL of Δ90CycB lysis buffer plus 8 M urea and 5 mM DTT, and incubate for 1 h at room temperature. Add 15 mL of Δ90CycB refolding buffer dropwise and centrifuge refolded Δ90CycB protein at 23,000g for 5 min at 4°C.
5. Dialyze cleared supernatant three times against Δ90CycB refolding buffer and concentrate by CentriPrep-10. We usually make a stock of Δ90CycB at 1 mg/mL.

3.2. Preparing Xenopus Extracts

Xenopus cell-free extracts are a powerful system to investigate the function of Chfr in the cell cycle. *Xenopus* laid eggs are normally arrested at meiotic metaphase II. Upon activation by calcium influx, eggs exit from meiosis and enter mitotic cycles. Cytoplasmic extracts can be easily prepared from activated eggs by a two-step centrifugation protocol, and such extracts cycle between interphase and mitosis multiple times in vitro. The following protocol is adapted from Murray et al. *(8)*.

3.2.1. Priming and Inducing Frogs to Lay Eggs

1. Prime frogs with pregnant mare serum gonadotropin (PMSG) 3 to 7 d prior to the day of your experiment. Inject each frog with 50 U of PMSG (100 U/mL) subcutaneously into the dorsal lymph sac using a 27-gage needle.
2. One day prior to your experiment, inject 500 U of human chorionic gonadotropin (hCG) (1000 U/mL) to induce ovulation. Place each frog in a 4-L container with 2 L of MMR and keep at 16°C overnight.

3.2.2. Preparing Cycling Extracts

1. Prepare 500 mL of MMR and 500 mL of XB per frog, and preequilibrate to 16°C.
2. Collect laid eggs 15–16 h after injection of hCG and wash eggs with MMR once (*see* **Note 4**).
3. Freshly prepare 200 mL of 2% cysteine, pH 7.6, per frog.
4. Dejelly eggs in 2% cysteine solution for 5 min. During this process, swirl eggs around gently to mix well. Dejellying is complete when eggs are closely packed and the volume of eggs is reduced to 20%.
5. Wash eggs with MMR three times, 100 mL per frog each time.
6. Activate eggs with 1 µg/mL of calcium ionophore (A23187) for 3–5 min. As soon as eggs become activated, the pigmented animal pole contracts. Do not overactivate (*see* **Note 5**).
7. Wash eggs with MMR once and with XB three times, 100 mL per frog each time.
8. Incubate activated eggs in XB for 20 min at room temperature. This incubation allows eggs to exit from metaphase arrest (*see* **Note 6**).
9. Set up 16 × 102 mm Beckman clear centrifuge tubes on ice and add 1 mL XB containing 10X protease inhibitor mix and 10X cytochalasin B to each tube.
10. Wash eggs once with small volume of ice-cold XB containing 1X protease inhibitor mix and transfer eggs to the centrifuge tubes prepared previously.
11. Aspirate off any excess buffer and add 1 mL of Nyosil-M25 oil to each tube (*see* **Note 7**).
12. Spin tubes at 2000*g* for 1 min in an HB-6 rotor to pack eggs.
13. Remove excess buffer and oil on top of tubes.
14. Crush eggs at 16,000*g* for 10 min at 4°C in a HB-6 rotor. During the centrifugation, set up a 3-mL syringe and 19-gage needle on ice to chill. Set up 13 × 51 mm Beckman clear centrifuge tubes and 17 × 100 mm polypropylene culture test tubes on ice for the second spin.
15. Collect the middle layer from tubes with needle and syringe. Place extracts in chilled Beckman tubes and add protease-inhibitor mix, cytochalasin B, and energy-regenerating system to 1X final concentrations. Insert the Beckman tube into the culture test tube.
16. Spin tubes at 8000*g* for 10 min at 4°C in the HB-6 rotor.
17. Collect the middle layer with a needle/syringe by poking on the side of tube and place extracts in chilled Eppendorf tubes. Use extracts immediately. Otherwise, add sucrose to 200 m*M* and freeze and store extracts at –80°C (*see* **Note 8**).

The yield of extracts is usually 0.5–1 mL per frog. Fresh extracts prepared with this protocol will cycle between interphase and mitosis two to three times once the temperature of extracts is raised to room temperature *(8)*. To generate interphase extracts, cycloheximide can be added to extracts at a final concentration of 10 mM to inhibit protein synthesis, and such extracts will stay at interphase. Interphase extracts can be induced to enter mitosis and arrest at anaphase upon addition of nondegradable Δ90CycB. Thus, the G2-to-M transition can be recapitulated by addition of Δ90CycB to interphase extracts *(8)*. Interphase and mitotic extracts can be frozen and stored at –80°C for 1 mo, but cycling extracts have to be prepared and used fresh.

3.3. Analyzing the Chfr Ubiquitin Ligase

3.3.1. Auto-Ubiquitination of Chfr

3.3.1.1. ASSAYING LIGASE ACTIVITY OF RECOMBINANT CHFR PROTEIN

As a ubiquitin ligase, Chfr auto-ubiquitinates in the presence of E1, E2, ubiquitin, and ATP, but in the absence of a substrate **(Fig. 1B)**. Auto-ubiquitination can be assayed in vitro as described here.

1. Label ubiquitin with ^{125}I to a specific activity of 100 μCi/μg using the chloramine T procedure *(9)*.
2. Perform auto-ubiquitination reactions in a total volume of 10 μL. The reaction mixture contains an energy-regenerating system, 400 μg/mL labeled ubiquitin, 20 μg/mL recombinant E1, 10 μg/mL Ubc4, and 800 μg/mL Chfr, Chfr1, Chfr2, or GST–Chfr3. Incubate reactions at room temperature for varying times and quench with SDS sample buffer.
3. Analyze reactions by reducing 12% SDS-PAGE and scan gels with a PhosphorImager.
   Through deletion analysis (ChfrF1-3), we found that the RF domain is sufficient for auto-ubiquitination activity **(Fig. 1C)**. In addition, point mutations in the RF domain (ChfrI306A and ChfrW332A) abolish the auto-ubiquitination activity. Thus, the RF domain is both necessary and sufficient for auto-ubiquitination activity.

3.3.1.2. ASSAYING LIGASE ACTIVITY OF CHFR FROM TRANSFECTED CELLS

The Chfr ligase activity can also be analyzed in mammalian tissue culture cells.

1. Transfect Myc–Chfr gene, Myc–ChfrI306A, and Myc–ChfrW332A (10 μg each) into HEK293T cells in a 10-cm dish using the calcium phosphate method. Harvest cells 72 h posttransfection.
2. Lyse cells with 500 μL of the HEK293T lysis buffer and sonicate lysates for 2 min. Centrifuge at 200,000g for 30 min at 4°C to make S100 supernatants.

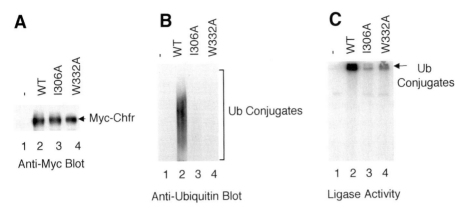

Fig. 2. The Chfr ligase activity from transfected cells. Myc–Chfr (lanes 2), Myc–ChfrI306A (lanes 3), Myc–ChfrW332A (lanes 4), and control vector (lanes 1) were transfected into HEK293T cells and immunoprecipitated by an anti-Myc antibody. The immunoprecipitates were analyzed by Western blotting with an anti-Myc antibody (**A**) or with an anti-ubiquitin antibody (**B**). In addition, immunoprecipitates were incubated with radioactive ubiquitin in the presence of recombinant E1 and Ubc4 and assayed for ubiquitin ligase activity (**C**).

3. Covalently couple the mouse anti-Myc antibody (9E10 clone) to Affi-Prep Protein A beads at a concentration of 1 µg of the antibody per µL of beads. Wash beads twice with 10 vol of 100 mM glycine, pH 2.5, to preelute uncrosslinked antibody, and then neutralize antibody beads with 10 mM Tris-HCl, pH 7.5.
4. Incubate 3 µL of antibody beads with 500 µL of S100 supernatant overnight at 4°C and mix antibody beads gently on a shaker. Wash antibody beads by gently mixing five times with 20 vol of XB buffer containing 500 mM KCl and 0.5% NP-40, and three times with XB alone. Elute proteins bound to beads with SDS sample buffer, separate eluted proteins by SDS-PAGE, and analyze by Western blotting using an anti-ubiquitin antibody (**Fig. 2A,B**).
5. For ubiquitination assays with Myc–Chfr complexes from HEK293T cells (**Fig. 2C**), transfect Myc–Chfr in a 15-cm dish of HEK293T cells. Purify Myc–Chfr by anti-Myc antibody beads and incubate anti-Myc immunoprecipitates in 5 µL with 400 µg/mL labeled ubiquitin, 20 µg/mL recombinant E1, 300 µg/mL Ubc4, and 1 mM ATP at room temperature for 1 h. Quench reactions with SDS sample buffer and analyze by reducing 10% SDS-PAGE.

3.3.2. Ubiquitinating the Chfr Substrate

Polo-like kinase, Plk1, is a substrate of Chfr at the G2/M transition. Plk1 phosphorylates Cdc25C phosphatase at the G2/M transition, leading to activation of Cdc2 and entry into mitosis. Ubiquitination and subsequent degradation of Plk1 by Chfr delays the activation of Cdc2 and mitotic entry.

Ubiquitination of Plk1 by Chfr can be demonstrated in vitro.

1. Synthesize Plk1 in a coupled transcription and translation reaction in reticulocyte lysates in the presence of [^{35}S]-Met.
2. Incubate labeled Plk1 with recombinant 20 μg/mL E1, 10 μg/mL Ubc4, 400 μg/mL Chfr, 400 μg/mL ubiquitin, and an energy-regenerating system at room temperature for varying times.
3. Quench reactions with SDS sample buffer and analyze by reducing 12% SDS-PAGE (**Fig. 3A**). Scan gels with a PhosphorImager. Formation of Plk1–Ub conjugates were detected in a Chfr-dependent manner (**Fig. 3A**).

Formation of the Plk1–Ub conjugates can be detected in *Xenopus* extracts.

1. Incubate recombinant GST-Ub protein (1 mg/mL) with *Xenopus* interphase extracts with or without recombinant Chfr (400 μg/mL) for 30 min at 4°C.
2. Add glutathione beads (2 μL bead/10 μL extracts) to the extracts and incubate for varying times at 4°C.
3. Collect aliquots of extracts with glutathione beads in cold XB buffer at various time points and purify GST–Ub conjugates by glutathione beads.
4. Detect conjugates of GST–Ub and Plx1 (the *Xenopus* homolog of Plk1) by Western blot analysis using an antibody against Plx1 (**Fig. 3B**). The formation of Plx1–GST–Ub conjugates depends on the addition of Chfr ligase.

Chfr-dependent degradation of Plx1 at G2/M transition can be monitored in *Xenopus* extracts, since entry into mitosis in this cell-free system can be induced by addition of nondegradable Δ90CycB to interphase extracts.

1. Incubate *Xenopus* interphase extracts with 2 mg/mL ubiquitin either in the presence or absence of 400 μg/mL recombinant Chfr.
2. Add Δ90CycB to 50 μg/mL and take aliquots of extracts at various time points. Detect the formation and degradation of Plx1–Ub conjugates kinetically by Western blot analysis using an antibody against Plx1 (**Fig. 3C**).

At the G2/M transition, active Chfr ligase mediates the formation of Plx1–Ub conjugates in *Xenopus* extracts, leading to the degradation of Plx1.

3.3.3. Effect of Chfr Ligase on Entry into Mitosis

Xenopus extracts are an excellent system to study the biological function of Chfr on cell-cycle progression, since this cell-free system can cycle between interphase and mitosis in vitro.

1. Incubate recombinant Chfr at 400 μg/mL with *Xenopus* cycling extracts.
2. Take 2 μL of extracts at various time points by quickly freezing in liquid nitrogen.
3. When all the samples are collected, measure the Cdc2 kinase activity using histone H1 as a substrate in 10 μL of EB buffer in the presence of radioactive γ-ATP. Assay reaction products by 12% SDS-PAGE and analyze by PhosphorImager (**Fig. 4A**).

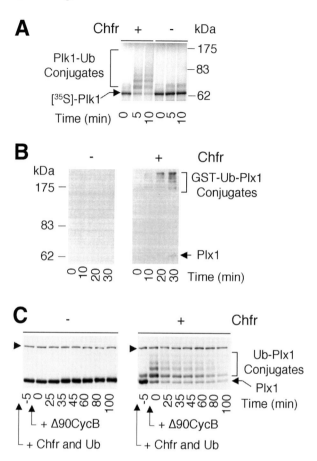

Fig. 3. Ubiquitination of Plk1 by the Chfr ligase. (**A**) In vitro ubiquitination of Plk1. In vitro-synthesized Plk1 was incubated with recombinant E1, Ubc4, ubiquitin, and ATP, either in the presence or absence of recombinant Chfr, and ubiquitination of Plk1 was analyzed by SDS-PAGE. (**B**) Isolation of Plx1–ubquitin conjugates from *Xenopus* extracts. *Xenopus* interphase extracts were incubated with GST–Ub plus a buffer or Chfr. Samples were collected at various time points and GST–Ub conjugates were purified with glutathione beads and assayed by Western blot analysis using the anti-Plx1 antibody. (**C**) Degradation of endogenous Plx1 at the G2/M transition in a Chfr-dependent manner. *Xenopus* interphase extracts were incubated with recombinant ubiquitin (at 2 mg/mL) plus a buffer or Chfr for 5 min. Δ90CycB was then added and the level of endogenous Plx1 at the G2/M transition was assayed by Western blotting with an anti-Plx1 antibody. Arrowheads point to nonspecific, cross-reacting bands.

In control extracts without Chfr, extracts cycle between interphase and mitosis twice within the first 120 min, whereas the Chfr-treated extracts enter the first mitosis only after 130 min. Thus, Chfr ligase causes a profound cell cycle delay (**Fig. 4A**).

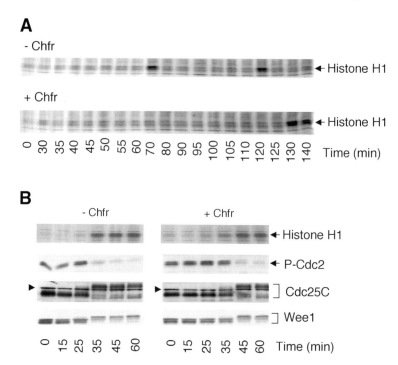

Fig. 4. Chfr controls the activation of Cdc2 at the G2-M transition. (**A**) *Xenopus* cycling extracts were incubated with either buffer (indicated as –Chfr) or Chfr and the kinetics of entry into mitosis were measured by the Cdc2 kinase activity assay using histone H1 as a substrate. (**B**) *Xenopus* interphase extracts were incubated with either buffer (–Chfr) or Chfr. Δ90CycB was then added and the activation of the Cdc2 kinase was determined. The kinetics of entry into mitosis were also measured by the phosphorylation state of Cdc2, Cdc25C, and Wee1 in Western blot analysis. Arrowheads point to nonspecific, cross-reacting bands.

To determine the exact cell cycle transition the Chfr pathway regulates, one can examine the G2 to M transition in detail by inducing the interphase to mitosis transition with addition of Δ90CycB to interphase extracts.

1. Incubate interphase extracts with recombinant Chfr at a final concentration of 400 μg/mL for 20 min.
2. Add Δ90CycB at a final concentration of 50 μg/mL. Take 1 μL samples at various time points by quickly freezing in liquid nitrogen.
3. When all the samples were collected, measure the Cdc2 kinase activity as described above (**Fig. 4B**). In addition, determine the level of Tyr-15 phosphorylated Cdc2 by Western blot analysis using an antibody specific to phosphorylated

Cdc2, but not to the unphosphorylated form. Determine the degrees of phosphorylation on Cdc25C phosphatase and on Wee1 kinase by their mobility shift on SDS-PAGE in Western blot analysis.

We conclude that active Chfr delays the entry into mitosis as measured by the activation of Cdc2 kinase at the G2/M transition. This delay correlates with the prolonged inhibitory phosphorylation on Tyr 15 of Cdc2. Consistent with this, active Chfr delays the phosphorylation of both Cdc25C and Wee1 at the G2/M transition (**Fig. 4B**).

Based on data presented here, we propose the following model for the Chfr pathway at the G2/M transition. During the normal G2/M transition, Wee1 mediates the inhibitory phosphorylation of Tyr 15 and Thr 14 on Cdc2, while Cdc25C dephosphorylates and activates Cdc2. Plk1 regulates both the Wee1 kinase and the Cdc25C phosphatase, which in turn control the Cdc2 kinase activity (**10**). Wee1 is phosphorylated by Plk1 as well as by Cdc2/cyclin B, and phosphorylation inhibits its kinase activity. On the other hand, the N-terminal regulatory domain in the Cdc25C protein is also phosphorylated by Plk1 and Cdc2/cyclin B. However, phosphorylation enhances the phosphatase activity of Cdc25C (**11–14**). Thus, the activation of Cdc25C and Cdc2 and the inhibition of Wee1 at mitosis constitute an auto-activating feedback loop that allows activation of the Cdc2 kinase in an all-or-none fashion (**10**). The initial activity of the Plk1 at the G2/M transition can determine the status of the auto-activating loop and the level of the Cdc2 kinase activity. Upon activation of the G2/M checkpoint, active Chfr ligase targets Plk1 for ubiquitination and degradation, leading to delayed activation of Cdc25C and Cdc2.

We expect that *Xenopus* extracts reflect certain aspects of regulation of Plk1 in mammalian somatic cells. The expression of Plk1 is regulated in mammalian cells; Plk1 begins to accumulate in G2 and its level peaks in mitosis (**15**). Activation of the Chfr pathway by mitotic stress leads to ubiquitination and degradation of Plk1 and blocks the entry into mitosis. Once mitotic stress is relieved and defects are repaired, the Chfr ligase is inactivated and *de novo* synthesis of Plk1 drives cells into mitosis. Thus, over-expression of Chfr in *Xenopus* extracts allows us to investigate checkpoint signaling from active Chfr to Cdc2. Using the *Xenopus* cell-free system, we have elucidated the molecular pathway leading from activation of Chfr to the delay in mitotic entry.

4. Notes

1. Chfr failed to express as a full-length recombinant protein in *E. coli*. When expressed in *Sf*9 cells, His–Chfr is soluble, but cannot be purified with Ni beads directly from cell lysates, presumably as a result of the inaccessibility of the His tag. However, we were able to quantitatively purify His–Chfr using Ni beads after prior fractionation of total cell lysates over a Resource Q anion exchange column.

2. ChfrF3 contains only the RF domain (93 amino acids). When expressed by itself in *E. coli*, no expression was detectable. Fusion of ChfrF3 to GST stabilizes the RF domain, leading to a high-level expression.

3. Although His-tagged E1 can be expressed in *E. coli* and purified by a Ni column, the purified prep contains a large number of truncated proteins. Purification by the Ni column tends to give a higher yield than that by the ubiquitin-affinity column. However, protein purified by Ni column is not active, presumably due to misfolding of E1 and the dominant-negative effect of the truncated proteins.

4. Frogs continue to lay eggs up to 24 h post hCG injection, but eggs tend to be less healthy after 20 h in MMR buffer. We usually collect eggs 16 h post hCG injection. To ensure the highest quality of laid eggs, it is important to pre-equilibrate MMR to 16°C and to keep frogs and eggs at 16°C all the time.

5. Prolonged incubation with calcium ionophore will cause extracts to fail to cycle and undergo apoptosis. It is critical to stop activation as soon as the animal pole begins to contract.

6. The 20 min incubation between activation and centrifugation ensures that meiotic regulators, such as c-mos, are completely down-regulated. Otherwise, extracts are able to cycle through interphase into mitosis, but fail to exit from mitosis.

7. Nyosil-M25 oil has a density higher than aqueous buffer, but lower than eggs. Upon low-speed packing centrifugation, Nyosil oil will sediment between eggs and the aqueous buffer, thereby allowing complete removal of buffer from eggs. For extracts to cycle, it is important to prepare extracts as concentrated as possible.

8. Sucrose stabilizes extracts. We usually add 200mM sucrose to interphase or mitotic extracts before freezing extracts and storing at –80°C. It is less important to include sucrose in cycling extracts, since cycling extracts are used immediately after preparation.

Acknowledgment

We are grateful to Drs. Bill Dunphy, Jim Ferrell, and James Maller for constructs and antibodies. J. W. is a recipient of the Howard Hughes Pre-doctoral Fellowship. G. F. is a Searle Scholar, a Kimmel Scholar in Cancer Research, and a recipient of the Beckman Young Investigator Award and the Burroughs-Wellcome Career Award in Biomedical Sciences. This work was also supported by an NIH R01 grant (GM62852) and by a Research Scholar Grant from the American Cancer Society (RSG-01-143-01).

References

1. Scolnick, D. M. and Halazonetis, T. D. (2000) Chfr defines a mitotic stress checkpoint that delays entry into metaphase. *Nature* **406**, 430–435.

2. Kang, D., Chen J., Wong, J., and Fang, G. (2002) The checkpoint protein Chfr is a ligase that ubiquitinates Plk1 and inhibits Cdc2 at the G2 to M transition. *J. Cell Biol.* **156**, 249–259.

3. Jha, M. N., Bamburg, J. R., and Bedford, J. S. (1994) Cell cycle arrest by Colcemid differs in human normal and tumor cells. *Cancer Res.* **54,** 5011–5015.

4. Mizuno, K., Osada, H., Konishi, H., et al. (2002) Aberrant hypermethylation of the CHFR prophase checkpoint gene in human lung cancers. *Oncogene* **21,** 2328–2333.

5. Shibata, Y., Haruki, N., Kuwabara, Y., et al. (2002) Chfr expression is downregulated by CpG island hypermethylation in esophageal cancer. *Carcinogenesis* **23,** 1695–1699.

6. Corn, P. G., Fogt, S. M., Virmani, F., Gazdar, A. K., Halazonetis, T. D., and El-Deiry, W. S. (2003) Frequent hypermethylation of the 5' CpG island of the mitotic stress checkpoint gene Chfr in colorectal and non-small cell lung cancer. *Carcinogenesis* **24,** 47–51.

7. Glotzer, M., Murray, A. W., and Kirschner, M. W. (1991) Cyclin is degraded by the ubiquitin pathway. *Nature* **349,** 132–138.

8. Murray, A. W. (1991) Cell cycle extracts. *Methods in Cell Biology* **36,** 581–605.

9. Parker, C. W. (1990) Radiolabeling of proteins. *Meth. Enzymol.* **182,** 721–737.

10. King, R. W., Jackson, P. K., and Kirschner, M. W. (1994) Mitosis in transition. *Cell* **79,** 563–571.

11. Izumi, T., Walker, D. H., and Maller, J. L. (1992) Periodic changes in phosphorylation of the *Xenopus* cdc25 phosphatase regulate its activity. *Mol. Biol. Cell* **3,** 927–939.

12. Izumi, T. and Maller, J. L. (1993) Elimination of cdc2 phosphorylation sites in the cdc25 phosphatase blocks initiation of M-phase. *Mol. Biol. Cell* **4,** 1337–1350.

13. Kumagai, A. and Dunphy, W. G. (1992) Regulation of the cdc25 protein during the cell cycle in *Xenopus* extracts. *Cell* **70,** 139–151.

14. Kumagai, A. and Dunphy, W. G. (1996) Purification and molecular cloning of Plx1, a Cdc25-regulatory kinase from *Xenopus* egg extracts. *Science* **273,** 1377–1380.

15. Fang, G., Yu, H., and Kirschner, M. W. (1998) Direct binding of CDC20 protein family members activates the anaphase-promoting complex in mitosis and G1. *Mol. Cell* **2,** 163–171.

11

Control of Mitotic Entry After DNA Damage in *Drosophila*

Burnley Jaklevic, Amanda Purdy, and Tin Tin Su

Summary

In the presence of DNA damage, cells delay the entry into mitosis, presumably to allow time for repair. Methods to detect the delay of mitosis in a multicellular model organism, *Drosophila melanogaster,* are described here. These include the collection of embryos and larvae, irradiation with x-rays to damage DNA, and fixing and staining of tissues with an antibody to phosphorylated histone H3 to measure the mitotic index. These methods should be useful in identifying potential mutants that are unable to regulate mitosis following DNA damage.

Key Words: *Drosophila;* embryo; larvae; cell cycle; mitosis; DNA damage; checkpoint.

1. Introduction

Cell proliferation is essential for growth and maintenance of all organisms. Equally important is the need to inhibit cell proliferation in response to extracellular and intracellular conditions such as the lack of nutrients or damaged and incompletely replicated DNA. Inability to regulate cell division in the presence of damaged DNA can compromise the genetic integrity of daughter cells. As such, mutational loss of checkpoint mechanisms that sense the presence of DNA defects and regulate the cell-division cycle as needed can increase genome instability and predisposition to cancer *(1)*. This chapter describes methods to assay for regulation of mitosis in the presence of damaged DNA in *Drosophila melanogaster.* Ionizing radiation (x-rays) is used to induce DNA damage, but the methods described here could also be used in combination with other DNA damaging radiation such as γ-rays and ultraviolet (UV). A commercially available antibody to a phosphorylated serine on histone H3 (PH3 *[2,3]*), a mitosis-specific antigen, is used to identify mitotic cells. These methods can be used to test potential checkpoint mutants for their ability to

From: *Methods in Molecular Biology, vol. 280: Checkpoint Controls and Cancer, Volume 1: Reviews and Model Systems*
Edited by: Axel H. Schönthal © Humana Press Inc., Totowa, NJ

regulate mitosis. Methods for detection of mitotic regulation in two different developmental stages, embryo and larvae, are described. Thus, maternal effect lethal or embryonic lethal mutants (i.e., when mutations prevent development beyond embryonic stages) can be assayed as embryos, while larval lethal mutants (i.e., when mutations permit development to larval stages) can be assayed at either stage. In summary, this chapter describes methods for collection of embryos and larvae, irradiation to induce DNA damage, and fixing and staining to detect changes in mitotic index.

2. Materials

1. Food for fly culture (*4–6*):
   a. Molasses agar bottles.
   b. Baker's yeast.
   c. Grape juice–agar plates.
2. Containers for fly culture:
   a. Collection cages—large plexiglass containers sealed at one end with insect screen. These hold flies during egg collection.
   b. Egg collection baskets—plexiglass cylinders sealed at one end with nylon netting.
3. A soft paint brush.
4. Small (35 × 10 mm) plastic petri dish.
5. Large (100 × 15 mm) plastic petri dish lid.
6. Two pair fine forceps, e.g., no. 5 Watchmaker.
7. Dissecting microscope.
8. Nutator or other rocking device to mix samples during incubation.
9. Phosphate buffered saline (PBS): 140 mM NaCl, 2.6 mM KCl, 10 mM Na$_2$HPO$_4$, 1.8 mM KH$_2$PO$_4$, pH 7.4.
10. Fix solution for larval tissues: 1X PBS, 5% formaldehyde, 0.3% Triton-X-100 (made fresh).
11. Fix solution for embryos: 1X PBS, 10% formaldehyde (made fresh).
12. PBTx: 1X PBS, 0.3% Triton-X-100.
13. Block solution; PBTx plus 10% Normal Goat Serum.
14. Rabbit anti-PH3 antibody (Upstate Biotech), diluted 1:1000 in block just prior to use.
15. Anti-rabbit secondary antibodies conjugated to FITC or rhodamine.
16. Flouromount-G (Southern Biotechnology Associates, Inc.).
17. Hoechst 33258 for staining DNA.
18. Microscope slides and coverslips.
19. Compound fluorescence microscope.
20. Heptane.
21. 50% bleach (made fresh in water).
22. Methanol.
23. X-ray source.

3. Methods

Subheadings 3.1.–3.4. apply to embryos and **Subheadings 3.5.–3.8.** apply to larvae. Methods outline (1) embryo collection and irradiation; (2) fixation; (3) staining to visualize mitotic cells; (4) data collection and interpretation; (5) collection and aging of embryos to reach appropriate larval stages; (6) irradiation; (7) dissection to obtain imaginal discs; and (8) fixation, staining, and interpretation of data.

3.1. Embryo Collection and Irradiation

A working knowledge of *Drosophila* culture is assumed but may be found in *(4,6)*. Flies and embryos are kept in a humidified incubator at 25°C throughout the procedure except for the brief interval needed for irradiation. Time intervals are adjusted for embryo development at 25°C and should be adhered to faithfully.

1. Collect embryos on a grape-agar plate for 60 min and discard (*see* **Note 1**). This precollection removes embryos that are abnormally older because adult females hold their eggs in the absence of fresh food. Next, use a fresh grape-agar plate to collect embryos for 10 min. These are the embryos you will use. Let embryos age for 325 min; this will allow cells of the dorsal epidermis to reach interphase of embryonic cell-division cycle 16 ((*7*); **Fig. 1**).
2. Cut the agar slab (with embryos) in half. Expose one half to 570 rads of x-rays, which is the LD$_{50}$ for this stage in embryogenesis; keep the other half, which serves as the unirradiated control, in the incubator (*see* **Note 2**).
3. Return irradiated embryos to the incubator and let experimental and control samples incubate for 10–20 min. The duration of this step depends on how fast the following steps can be performed. The key is to place embryos in the fix at exactly 20 min after irradiation.

3.2. Fixation

This step is carried out at room temperature (RT).

1. Squirt dH$_2$O onto embryos and loosen them from agar using a soft paint brush. Pour water with embryos into the egg collection basket and rinse with dH$_2$O to remove yeast. Blot with tissue paper to remove excess dH$_2$O.
2. Dechorionate embryos (remove the chorion) by placing basket in 50% bleach for 2 min. Swirl embryos occasionally. Remove basket and rinse embryos extensively with dH$_2$O to remove all bleach. Blot to remove excess dH$_2$O.
3. Transfer basket to a petri dish containing heptane. Prewet 1 mL plastic pipet tip by pipeting heptane up and down a few times; this prevents embryo from sticking to the side of pipet tips. Trim the end of the pipet tip to enlarge the opening; this prevents tissue damage. Use a Pipetman® to transfer embryos to 20-mL glass vial containing 3 mL of fix solution. Add 3 mL heptane to glass vial and rock the vial for 20 min at RT.

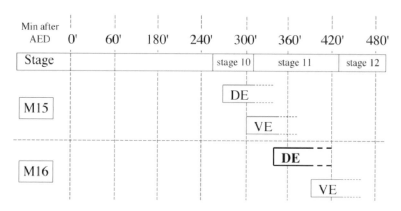

Fig. 1. Timetable for mitosis in embryonic cell cycle 15 and 16 (M15 and M16, respectively). The approximate time of mitotic entry for the dorsal and ventral epidermis (de and ve, respectively) is diagrammed. The time after egg deposition (AED) is shown for 25°C.

4. Remove most of the lower phase (aqueous fix layer). Add 10 mL MeOH to glass vial and shake vigorously for 30 s to remove the vitelline membrane that encloses the embryo. Let embryos settle (*see* **Note 3**).
5. MeOH and heptane will separate into two phases; embryos trapped at the interface did not lose the vitelline membrane and are not useful for antibody staining. Collect embryos only from the bottom of glass vial and transfer to a new microfuge tube. Wash embryos 3 times with MeOH. These can be stored at −20°C in MeOH for several months or processed for antibody staining directly.

3.3. Antibody Staining

All steps are performed at RT. Starting with **step 6**, samples should be kept in the dark by wrapping in foil.

1. Using a Pipetman with a cut off tip, transfer embryos to a new 1.5-mL microfuge tube. Remove excess MeOH.
2. Rehydrate embryos with three rinses of PBTx. Rock embryos in the last rinse for 5 min.
3. Replace the last PBTx rinse with block solution and incubate for at least 1 h while rocking.
4. Replace block solution with the primary antibody (1:1000 rabbit anti-PH3 in block) and rock for 2 h.
5. Wash three times for 15 min with block solution.
6. Add secondary antibody solution, diluted 1:500 in block solution, and rock for 2 h (*see* **Note 4**).
7. Wash three times for 15 min with PBTx.

8. Replace the last wash with 1 mL Hoechst solution (10 µg/mL in PBTx) and rock for 4 min.
9. Wash three times for 15 min with PBTx.
10. Mount embryos in Fluoromount-G and analyze.

3.4. Data Collection and Interpretation

1. Use a fluorescent microscope with a ×10 or 20 objective to identify embryos of the correct orientation and correct age. It is easiest to use Hoechst staining to identify morphological markers (**Fig. 2**).
2. Using a higher power objective (×40–100), quantify the total number of PH3-positive cells within the entire dorsal epidermis (de) of the embryo. It is easiest to begin counting mitotic cells just below the last gnathal lobe (gl) and continue around the amnioserosa to include the entire dorsal epidermis (**Figs. 2 and 3**).
3. Count at least 10 embryos each from unirradiated and irradiated samples. Wild-type embryos typically show about 85% reduction in mitotic index at 20 min after irradiation (reduction from 111 ±14 to 17 ±11 mitotic cells in **Fig. 3**).

3.5. Collecting and Aging to Obtain Third Instar Larvae

A working knowledge of fly culture is assumed but may be found in *(4,6)*.

1. Place *Drosophila* adults in a molasses agar bottle seeded with yeast and allow egg deposition for 2–4 h; adjust collection time to avoid a high density of embryos (*see* **Note 5**).
2. Remove adults from bottle.
3. Age embryos for 4 d at 25°C to reach late third instar stage of larval development, during which larvae crawl out of the food and up the bottle wall (*see* **Note 6**).

3.6. Irradiation

In wild-type larvae, inhibition of mitosis is apparent at 1 h after irradiation in both wing and eye-antennal imaginal discs *(8)*. This is because cells in mitosis at the time of irradiation have exited mitosis, and further entry into mitosis is prevented by irradiation. Mitoses resume by 6 h after irradiation, indicating that the activation of the DNA damage checkpoint is transient.

1. Use a soft paintbrush wetted with water to transfer larvae into a petri dish containing water (*see* **Note 7**).
2. Irradiate larvae in petri dish with 4000 rads of x-rays, which is the LD_{50} for this stage in development (*see* **Note 8**).
3. Allow larvae to recover at 25°C. The recovery time will depend on how fast the following dissection steps can be performed. The key is to be able to incubate tissues in fix solution by 1 h after irradiation.

3.7. Dissection

This step is performed at room temperature. During fixing and staining, larval tissues remain in microfuge tubes. To prevent tissue loss, allow adequate

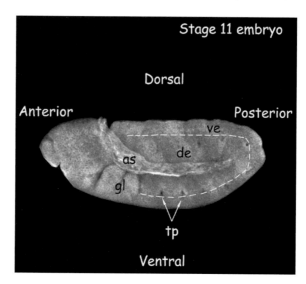

Fig. 2. Stage 11 embryo. This embryo was stained with Texas Red–conjugated Wheat Germ Agglutinin (Molecular Probes) to visualize major morphological markers. The dorsal and ventral epidermis (de and ve, respectively) are marked. The gnathal lobes (gl) and trachael pits (tp) are characteristic of this stage embryo. as = amnioserosa. Embryo staging is as in *(13)*.

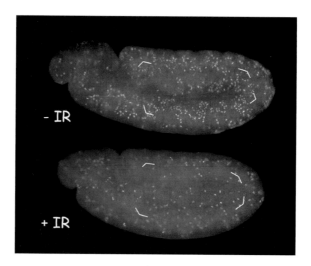

Fig. 3. Stage 11 embryos were irradiated with 0 (–IR) or 570 rad (+IR) of x-rays before fixing and staining with an anti-PH3 antibody to visualize mitotic cells. Quantification of PH3-stained cells in the dorsal epidermis (shown enclosed by brackets) from similar embryos show a reduction in mitoses in irradiated embryos.

time for tissues to settle to bottom of tubes and use a Pipetman instead of vacuum aspiration to remove all solutions.

1. Place larvae in a drop of PBS on the underside of a petri plate lid.
2. Extricate imaginal discs. This is best done by first grabbing the protruding mouth hooks with one pair of forceps and holding the larva approximately two-thirds down the body length with the other pair of forceps. Once forceps are in place, pull the mouthhooks away from the larval body. In addition to the translucent imaginal discs, salivary glands, optic lobes, fat, and the gut will come out attached to the mouthhooks (**Fig. 4** *[9]*). Use forceps to remove salivary glands, fat, and gut tissue. Eye-antennal imaginal discs sit atop the optic lobes and are attached via the optic nerve stalk; leave all attached to mouthhooks. Use forceps to grab mouthhooks and transfer tissues to a fresh drop of PBS.
3. Using this method of dissection, it is difficult to consistently obtain wing discs. Another method of dissection more conducive to obtaining wing discs involves pinching the larvae in half with forceps, then turning the anterior portion of the larvae inside out by using forceps to push the anterior mouth hooks through the new opening.
4. Repeat to obtain imaginal discs from 5 to 10 larvae.

3.8. Fixation and Staining

1. Transfer all dissected tissues to a 1.5-mL microfuge tube containing 1 mL fixing solution. Gently rock for 20 min.
2. Allow tissues to settle to the bottom and use a pipet to remove fix solution (*see* **Note 9**). Wash for 10 min with 1 mL of PBTx while gently rocking. Repeat the washing step twice (*see* **Note 10**).
3. Replace wash solution with the primary antibody (rabbit anti-PH3 diluted 1:1000 in block solution; at least 300 µL/tube); incubate at 4°C for 12 or more h with rocking.
4. Replace the primary antibody with 1 mL PBTx and wash for 10 min with rocking. Repeat wash twice.
5. Dilute secondary antibody 1:500 in block solution (*see* **Note 4**). Add at least 300 µL/tube and incubate for at least 2 h at RT. Remove and discard secondary antibody. This and all subsequent incubation steps are carried out in the dark by wrapping samples in foil.
6. Replace secondary antibody solution with 1 mL PBTx and wash for 10 min with rocking. Repeat wash twice.
7. Add 1 mL of PBTx with 10 µg/mL of Hoescht 33528 and incubate for 2 min with rocking.
8. Replace Hoechst solution with 1 mL PBTx and wash for 5 min with rocking. Repeat twice.
9. To mount tissues onto microscope slide, use a wide-mouthed 200-µL pipet tip to withdraw a mouth hook with attached discs and place on microscope slide.
10. Remove most of PBTx on slide using a pipet.

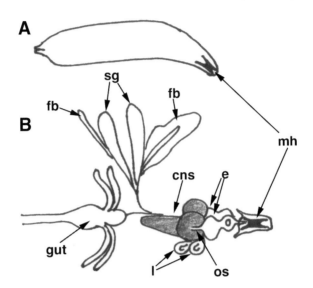

Fig. 4. Schematic representation of a third instar larva (**A**) and larval tissues (**B**): mh = mouthhooks; sg = salivary glands; fb = fat body; cns = central nervous system (optic lobes and ventral nerve cord, shaded); os= optic nerve stalk; e = eye-antennae imaginal disc; l = leg imaginal disc. Only two representative masses of fat body are shown.

11. Drop 50 µL of Flourmount-G onto tissues. Use forceps or tungsten needles to pull eye-antennal and wing discs away from the other tissues. To free eye-antennal discs, sever the optic stalk, which attaches each eye-antennal disc to each optic lobe of the brain. This step needs to be performed quickly because Flourmount-G will thicken fast.
12. Cover with coverslip and seal with clear fingernail polish.
13. Image discs using a compound fluorescence microscope. The eye-antennal and wing discs are sac-like epithelial structures that are comprised of two cell layers: an apical peripodial layer composed of large squamous cells, and a basal columnar layer (*10,11*). The columnar cells contribute to adult structures, but peripodial cells do not contribute to the adult. Both cell types show inhibition of mitosis after DNA damage. Thus, the number of mitotic cells showing PH3 stain can be quantified for the whole disc and compared with irradiated and non-irradiated larvae (*see* **Notes 11** and **12**).

4. Notes

1. Several drops of yeast paste in water are placed onto grape-agar plates to induce egg laying. Yeast paste should be blotted dry with a paper towel in order to prevent flies from sticking to it.
2. If the x-ray generator has not been properly calibrated, Lethal Dose 50 (LD$_{50}$) should be empirically determined for an individual x-ray machine as "the dose

that yields 50% mortality." LD_{50} for various developmental stages of *Drosophila* can be found in *(4)*.

3. When adding MeOH at the end of fixation, make sure there is still a heptane layer; this helps to trap embryos that did not lose their vitelline membrane at the interface. If there is not a discrete heptane layer, add 1–2 mL of heptane and shake for 30 s; this should restore the heptane layer. It is possible to lose up to 50% of embryos at the interface between MeOH and heptane during the fixation step.

4. Secondary antibodies are preabsorbed to remove nonspecifically binding antibodies. This is done by diluting the secondary antibody in block solution at 1:10 and incubating with an equal volume of fixed embryos for at least 2 h. The antibody solution is then removed and stored in a separate tube for up to 6 mo. It should be diluted 50-fold just before use to give a working dilution of 1:500.

5. Sparse embryo collections might result from adults either too young or old. Conversely, competition for resources will slow *Drosophila* development such that few larvae will be in the wandering stage on d 4. To avoid overcrowded conditions, adjust embryo collection time based on female fecundity, or use a spatula to transfer a small section of agar along with embryos to a new bottle.

6. At 25°C, the wandering third instar larval stage lasts approx 24 h and is followed by pupariation, where larvae become immobile. Third instar larvae undergoing pupariation will move slowly and should be avoided if dissecting eye-antennal discs to assay for the mitotic checkpoint. Eye-antennal discs from older animals begin folding and are difficult to image.

7. Oxygen deprivation (hypoxia) can halt cell cycle proliferation; take care not to submerge larvae in water during and after irradiation. Easy to recognize, hypoxic larvae move sluggishly and die if unable to move from water. Conversely, crawling third instar larvae move rapidly, and care should be taken to prevent escape, which might ensue if there is too little water in the petri dish.

8. LD_{50} for various developmental stages of *Drosophila* can be found in *(4)*. Always irradiate wild-type larvae along with mutant larvae to control for a functional x-ray source.

9. Problems with antibody staining (i.e., little or no signal) can often be traced back to over-fixing. Remove fix promptly.

10. Imaginal tissues are incredibly fragile. After fixation, tissues can be left at 4°C for up to 24 h if necessary; incubating longer can lead to excessive tissue degradation. If at all possible, antibody staining should begin immediately after fixation.

11. Detailed description of imaginal discs can be found in *(4)*. Both the eye-antennal disc and the wing disc are large, easy to identify, and useful in assaying for the mitotic checkpoint. These discs contribute to the *Drosophila* adult by forming the eye-antennae and the wing, respectively, during metamorphosis. During third instar larval development, eye-antennal discs have a well defined region of mitotic cells posterior to the morphogenetic furrow (**Fig. 5;** *(12)*), as well as asynchronous mitoses. Wing disc mitoses occur randomly during the larval third instar. The wing imaginal disc is loosely attached to the cluster of imaginal discs

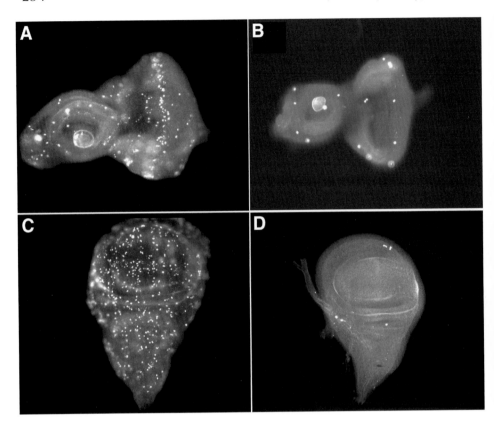

Fig. 5. Mitoses in eye-antennal and wing discs with and without irradiation. All imaginal discs have been incubated with an antibody against PH3 to detect cells in mitosis. (**A,B**) Eye-antennal and (**C,D**) wing imaginal discs from larvae that were not irradiated (**A,C**), or irradiated with 4000 rads of x-rays (**B,D**) and allowed to recover for 1 h.

and brain that leave the body with the mouthhooks, and is easily lost during dissection and subsequent incubation steps. Allowing ample time for tissues to settle to the bottom of the tube helps prevent the loss of wing discs. The eye-antennal disc, on the other hand, which is attached to the brain and the mouthhooks, is difficult to lose.

12. If the background fluorescence is too high, try incubating larval tissues in block solution for 1 h before adding primary antibody, or reduce the amount of time the tissues are in secondary antibody. If the signal is too low, try incubating tissues in primary antibody overnight at room temperature instead of 4°C.

Acknowledgments

We thank Maria Pagratis and Mark Robida for critical reading of the manuscript, and Anita Wichmann for technical assistance with **Fig. 5**. Work in the Su lab is supported by grants from the American Cancer Society (RPG-99-166-01-CCG) and the National Institutes of Health (RO1-GM66441). A. P. and B. R. J. are supported by a NIH pre-doctoral training grant.

References

1. Zhou, B. B. and Elledge, S. J. (2000) The DNA damage response: putting checkpoints in perspective. *Nature* **408,** 433–439.
2. Hendzel, M. J., Wei, Y., Mancini, M. A., et al. (1997) Mitosis-specific phosphorylation of histone H3 initiates primarily within pericentromeric heterochromatin during G2 and spreads in an ordered fashion coincident with mitotic chromosome condensation. *Chromosoma* **106,** 348–360.
3. Su, T. T., Sprenger, F., DiGregorio, P. J., Campbell, S. D., and O'Farrell, P. H. (1998) Exit from mitosis in *Drosophila* syncytial embryos requires proteolysis and cyclin degradation, and is associated with localized dephosphorylation. *Genes Dev.* **12,** 1495–1503.
4. Ashburner, M. (1989) *Drosophila: A Laboratory Handbook.* Cold Spring Harbor Laboratory, Cold Spring Harbor, NY.
5. Sullivan, W., Ashburner, M., and Hawley, R. S., eds. (2000) Appendix 3. In: *Drosophila Protocols.* Cold Spring Harbor Laboratory, Cold Spring Harbor, NY: pp. 655–659.
6. Sisson, J. C. (2000) Culturing large populations of *Drosophila* for protein biochemistry. In: *Drosophila Protocols* (Sullivan, W., Ashburner, M., and Hawley, R. S., eds.). Cold Spring Harbor Laboratory, Cold Spring Harbor, NY: pp. 541–551.
7. Foe, V. E., Odell, G. M., and Edgar, B. A. (1993) Mitosis and morphogenesis in the *Drosophila* embryo. In: *The Development of Drosophila melanogaster* (Bate, M. and Martinez Arias, A., eds.). Cold Spring Harbor Laboratory, Cold Spring Harbor, NY: pp. 149–300.
8. Brodsky, M. H., Sekelsky, J. J., Tsang, G., Hawley, R. S., and Rubin, G. M. (2000) *mus304* encodes a novel DNA damage checkpoint protein required during *Drosophila* development. *Genes Dev.* **14,** 666–678.
9. Wolff, T. (2000) Histological techniques for the *Drosophila* eye. Part I: Larva and pupa. In: *Drosophila Protocols* (Sullivan, W., Ashburner, M., and Hawley, R. S., eds). Cold Spring Harbor Laboratory, Cold Spring Harbor, NY: pp. 201–227.
10. Fristrom, D. and Fristrom, J. W. (1993) The metamorphic development of the adult epidermis. In: *The Development of Drosophila melanogaster* (Bate, M. and Martinez Arias, A., eds). Cold Spring Harbor Laboratory, Cold Spring Harbor, NY: pp. 843–897.

11. Wolff, T. and Ready, D. F. (1993) Pattern formation in the *Drosophila* retina. In: *The Development of Drosophila melanogaster* (Bate, M. and Martinez Arias, A., eds). Cold Spring Harbor Laboratory, Cold Spring Harbor, NY: pp. 1277–1326.

12. Thomas, B. J., Gunning, D. A., Cho, J., and Zipursky, L. (1994) Cell cycle progression in the developing *Drosophila* eye: *roughex* encodes a novel protein required for the establishment of G1. *Cell* **77,** 1003–1014.

13. Campos-Ortega, J. A. and Hartenstein, V. (1985) *The Embryonic Development of Drosophila melanogaster*. Springer-Verlag, Berlin.

12

Methods for Analyzing Checkpoint Responses in *Caenorhabditis elegans*

Anton Gartner, Amy J. MacQueen, and Anne M. Villeneuve

Summary

In response to genotoxic insults, cells activate DNA damage checkpoint pathways that stimulate DNA repair, lead to a transient cell cycle arrest, and/or elicit programmed cell death (apoptosis) of affected cells. The *Caenorhabditis elegans* germ line was recently established as a model system to study these processes in a genetically tractable, multicellular organism. The utility of this system was revealed by the finding that upon treatment with genotoxic agents, premeiotic *C. elegans* germ cells transiently halt cell cycle progression, whereas meiotic prophase germ cells in the late pachytene stage readily undergo apoptosis. Further, accumulation of unrepaired meiotic recombination intermediates can also lead to the apoptotic demise of affected pachytene cells. DNA damage-induced cell death requires key components of the evolutionarily conserved apoptosis machinery. Moreover, both cell cycle arrest and pachytene apoptosis responses depend on conserved DNA damage checkpoint proteins. Genetics- and genomics-based approaches that have demonstrated roles for conserved checkpoint proteins have also begun to uncover novel components of these response pathways. In this chapter, we will briefly review the *C. elegans* DNA damage-response field, and we will discuss in detail the methods that are being used to assay DNA damage responses in *C. elegans*.

Key Words: *C. elegans*; *C. elegans* germ line; *C. elegans* methods; apoptosis; programmed cell death; DNA damage responses; *ced* genes; germ line; checkpoint responses; p53; *cep-1*; cell cycle arrest; RNAi; RNAi feeding; co-suppression; meiosis; recombination.

1. Introduction

The correct maintenance and duplication of genetic information is constantly challenged by genotoxic stress. Such stress may result from exogenous insults, such as exposure to ionizing radiation or genotoxic chemicals, or may arise by endogenous means—e.g., mistakes in DNA replication, or oxidative damage as a result of intracellular reactive oxygen species. In response to genotoxic

From: *Methods in Molecular Biology, vol. 280: Checkpoint Controls and Cancer, Volume 1: Reviews and Model Systems*
Edited by: Axel H. Schönthal © Humana Press Inc., Totowa, NJ

stress, cells activate checkpoint pathways that lead to (1) DNA repair; (2) a transient cell cycle arrest in order to allow for time to repair compromising genetic lesions; or (3) apoptosis to trigger the demise of genetically damaged cells that might potentially become harmful to the entire organism.

1.1. Organization of the Nematode Germ Line

To investigate DNA damage-induced apoptosis and cell cycle arrest in a multicellular, genetically tractable model organism, we began to employ the germ line of the nematode worm *Caenohrabditis elegans* as an experimental system *(1)*. In contrast to classical studies of apoptosis in *C. elegans* that examined developmentally programmed, somatic cell deaths, DNA damage responses are best studied in the germ line, which is the only proliferative tissue in the adult worm. The germ line proliferates both during larval development and adulthood, and comprises about half of the cell nuclei in the adult worm *(2)*. The adult hermaphrodite gonad consists of two separate arms, each with a tubular structure. Throughout most of the length of each gonad arm, germ cell nuclei are present in a monolayer at the periphery of this tube, partially separated from each other by plasma membranes but retaining access to a common syncytial cytoplasmic core known as the rachis *(2)*. Further, germ cells are organized in a temporal/spatial gradient along the distal-proximal axis **(Fig. 1)**. The most distal end of the germ line contains a mitotic stem cell compartment, which is followed by nuclei in premeiotic S phase and progressively later substages of meiotic prophase; the most abundant group of meiotic cells are in the pachytene stage, during which homologous chromosomes are fully aligned and synapsed. The simultaneous presence of germ cells at different cell cycle and developmental stages indicates that adjacent germ cells are substantially insulated from their neighbors despite the syncytial organization of the germ line *(2)*.

1.2. Programmed Cell Death in the C. elegans Germ Line

Two key findings paved the way for using the nematode germ line to investigate DNA damage checkpoint responses. The first crucial observation was that programmed cell death in *C. elegans* occurs not only in the developmentally determined somatic cell lineages, but also in the germ lines of hermaphrodite worms *(3)*. Gumienny et al. noticed the presence of approx 0–4 germ cell corpses at any given time in the late pachytene region in the germ lines of normal adult hermaphrodites *(3)*. The first morphologically visible step of programmed cell death in the germ line is the complete cellularization of the cell that is destined to die; other stages closely resemble programmed cell deaths that occur during somatic development.

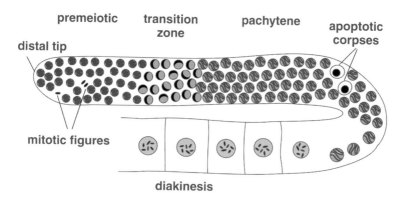

Fig. 1. Spatial organization of the *C. elegans* adult hermaphrodite germ line. Diagram shows one gonad arm, with individual germ line nuclei represented by black and gray circles; black areas represent the approximate appearance of chromatin as visualized by DAPI staining. The region adjacent to the distal tip contains premeiotic germ line nuclei, most of which are continuing to undergo mitotic cell cycles (mitotic figures are indicated); nuclei just distal to the "transition zone" region are in premeiotic S phase. Nuclei enter meiotic prophase in the transition zone, where a major nuclear reorganization that coincides with homologous chromosome pairing results in clustering of chromosomes toward one side of the nucleus; this organization imparts a crescent-shaped appearance to the DAPI-stained chromatin. The transition zone is followed by nuclei at the pachytene stage of meiotic prophase, in which chromosomes are organized in parallel pairs and are widely dispersed about the periphery of each nucleus. Apoptotic cell corpses (indicated by larger ovals with compact DAPI signals) are typically located in the late pachytene region, near to the bend of the gonad arm. Oocyte nuclei in diakinesis, the last stage of meiotic prophase, have greatly enlarged nuclei, and chromosome pairs have become highly condensed.

Within the germ line, only cells in the late pachytene stage of oocyte meiotic prophase are competent to die by apoptosis. Because dead cells are removed by phagocytosis, only a small number of dying cells or cell corpses will be visible at any given time; however, it has been estimated that as many as half of all potential oocyte precursors may be eliminated by programmed cell death during the reproductive life of an adult hermaphrodite. Since these deaths occur apparently independently of environmental stimuli, they have been termed "physiological" germ cell deaths. Similar to somatic apoptosis, physiological germ cell death is dependent on *ced-3* and *ced-4*, which encode the homologs of mammalian caspases and Apaf-1, respectively, and is suppressed by a gain-of-function mutation in Bcl2 ortholog *ced-9*. Further, the engulfment of germ cell corpses requires the same machinery used for engulfment during somatic cell death. However, the somatic cell death trigger *egl-1* is not required for physiological germ cell death *(3)*.

1.3. Germ Line Responses to Ionizing Radiation

A second key finding was that genotoxic stresses such as ionizing radiation (IR) can induce elevated levels of programmed cell death in the *C. elegans* germ line *(1)*. Upon irradiation, *C. elegans* germ cells activate checkpoint pathways that lead to either a transient cell cycle arrest or to programmed cell death (**Figs. 2** and **3**). These two DNA damage responses are spatially separated within the gonad: whereas germ cells in the mitotic region halt cell cycle progression, germ cells in the late pachytene region undergo apoptosis. Cells outside the germ line show neither of these responses *(1)*.

As is the case for physiological germ cell death, radiation-induced apoptosis appears to be restricted to female germ cells, requires *ced-3* (caspase) and *ced-4 (Apaf4)*, and is suppressed by a *ced-9 (Bcl2)* gain-of-function mutation *(1)*. Unlike physiological germ cell deaths, however, radiation-induced apoptosis is partially dependent on *egl-1*. The DNA-damage checkpoint can be activated not only by exogenous genotoxic insults, but also by meiotic defects that result in accumulation of unrepaired meiotic recombination intermediates. As part of the normal meiotic program, double-strand DNA breaks (DSBs) are generated by the meiotic endonuclease SPO-11 to initiate meiotic recombination *(4)*. These DSBs are resected to generate single-strand 3' overhangs, which invade the DNA duplex on the homolgous chromosome via a reaction mediated by the conserved RAD-51 strand-exchange protein. Worms lacking RAD-51 are thought to accumulate unrepaired resected DSBs, which are recognized at least in part by the very same checkpoint pathways that sense radiation-induced DSBs, thereby triggering elevated levels of germ cell apoptosis *(1,5)*.

In the mitotically proliferating region of the germ line, a transient halt in cell cycle progression is the second defining output of checkpoint activation *(1)*. Under normal growth conditions, the total number of syncytial germ cell nuclei increases steadily over time. After ionizing irradiation, however, the number of germ cell nuclei does not increase over a time window of 12 h as cell proliferation is transiently halted (**Fig. 3**). In addition to arrest of cell proliferation, the volume of mitotic germ cell nuclei as well as their surrounding cytoplasm becomes greatly enlarged following irradiation (**Fig. 3**), presumably because cellular and nuclear growth continues during radiation-induced cell-proliferation arrest. This phenomenon parallels classical descriptions of cell cycle arrest phenotypes in yeast and *Drosophila* systems *(6,7)*.

1.4. Germ Line Responses to Replication Block

Hydroxyurea (HU) depletes cellular dNTP pools through its specific inhibition of ribonucleotide reductase, and thus has been widely used as a potent

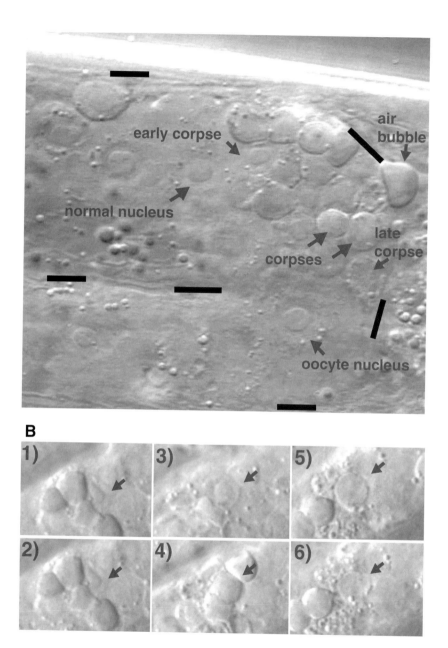

Fig. 2. Morphology of apototic germ cell corpses. (A) Example of massive germ cell death at the bend of the germ line. The morphologies of normal pachytene-stage meiotic prophase nuclei and of "early corpses," "corpses," and "late corpses" are indicated by arrows. (B) Time course of programmed germ cell death, following the fate of a dying cell over a period of approx 1.5 h. The arrow in each panel indicates the same cell at progressively later time points. Adapted from *(1)*.

0 Gy   **120 Gy**

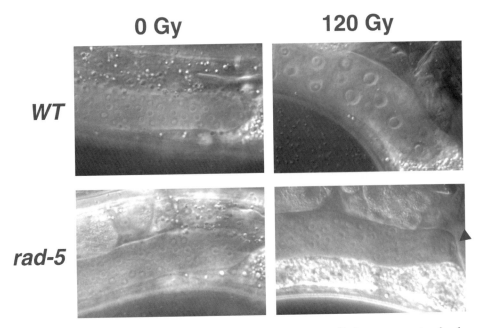

Fig. 3. Proliferation arrest phenotype of mitotic germ cells in response to check-point activation by IR, viewed with Nomarski microscopy. Note the enlargement of nuclei and the surrounding cytoplasm in response to irradiation in the WT animal. Checkpoint-defective animals like *rad-5* worms do not respond to ionizing irradiation. The arrowhead points to the distal tip cell.

indirect inhibitor of DNA synthesis. Numerous studies using HU to inhibit DNA replication have uncovered evidence for a checkpoint that monitors S phase progression in eukaryotic cells (*8–10*). Not surprisingly, chronic exposure of mature *C. elegans* hermaphrodites to HU elicits a block to germ cell proliferation, presumably as a consequence of inhibiting DNA replication (*11*). Compared with untreated control germ lines, HU-treated germ lines that have been stained with DAPI to label DNA (1) lack condensed mitotic figures representing nuclei undergoing M phase of the cell cycle; and (2) contain a reduced density of oversized nuclei with abnormally diffuse DAPI signals in their premeiotic regions (**Fig. 4B**). Both in DAPI-stained preparations and when viewed

Fig. 4. *(opposite page)* Assessment of HU-induced germ cell proliferation arrest. (**A**) Quantitation of numbers of germ cell nuclei in wild-type and *chk-2* mutant worms chronically exposed to HU, compared with untreated controls. Germ line nuclei in "optically bisected" gonad arms were counted 12 or 24 h after initiating the exposure of L4 larvae to 25 m*M* HU. Each data point represents the average value from 4 to 10 germ lines; error bars indicate standard deviations. Whereas germ cell numbers increased substantially between the 12- and 24-h time points in untreated control germ lines, no increase in numbers was observed in HU-treated germ lines, indicating arrest

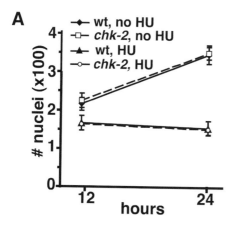

A

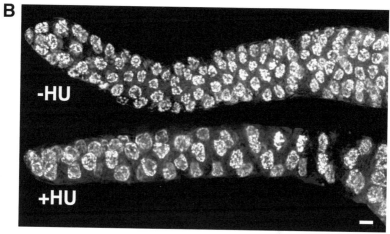

B

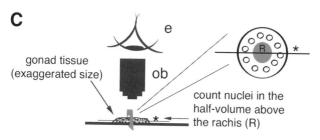

C

of germ cell proliferation; this checkpoint response was not abrogated in the *chk-2* mutant. (**B**) Morphological changes in premeiotic nuclei of *chk-2* mutants after 12 h of HU exposure; the response of wild-type germ lines is identical. Shown is the distal germ line region, which primarily contains premeiotic nuclei. In HU-treated germ lines, nuclei are substantially enlarged, reduced in number, and DAPI signals appear abnormally diffuse. Bar, 4 μm. (**A**) and (**B**) are reprinted with permission from *(11)*. (**C**) Diagram illustrating "optical bisection" of the germ line. The nucleus-free core (rachis) of the germ line is depicted in gray in the enlarged cross-section (R). The straight line bisecting the germ line at the midpoint along the Z axis represents the lower boundary for counting; nuclei in the half-volume of the germ line at or above this line should be included in counts. (e), observer eye, (ob), objective lens.

by Nomarski microscopy in live animals, the appearance of nuclei in the pre-meiotic region of HU-treated germ lines is reminiscent of that exhibited by premeiotic nuclei arrested by ionizing radiation (*[12]* and AJM, unpublished results). Germ line nuclei already in meiotic prophase appear largely unaffected by HU treatment.

HU-induced cell cycle arrest in *C. elegans* germ line nuclei appears to be reversible in a majority of affected germ cells, since mitotic figures reappear and many premeiotic nuclei exhibit normal size and morphology by 24 h after removal from HU (AJM, unpublished). Even 36 h following removal from HU, however, a handful of nuclei continue to exhibit arrest morphology. The apparent inability of a subset of nuclei to recover from arrest might reflect general cellular toxicity of the HU treatment, or it might reflect a difference between nuclei that were in S phase vs other phases of the cell cycle when dNTPs were depleted below critical levels. Alternatively, there might be differences in recovery potential between nuclei that were in pre-meiotic S phase at the time of depletion and those still undergoing proliferative cell cycles.

1.5. C. elegans *Checkpoint Genes and Checkpoint Responses*

Screens for *C. elegans* mutants defective in DNA-damage-induced apoptosis lead to the identification of *mrt-2, rad-5,* and *hus-1* as genes encoding potential checkpoint components *(1,12,13)*. Mutations in these genes result in abrogation of IR-induced cell-cycle arrest and resistance to IR-induced apoptosis, and render the worms hypersensitive to DNA damage. *mrt-2* was found not only to be required for the DNA-damage checkpoint but also for the regulation of telomere replication *(14)*. Positional cloning revealed that *mrt-2* encodes the worm ortholog of the *Schizzosaccharomyces pombe rad1* and *Saccharomyces cerevisiae rad17* checkpoint genes. *rad1/rad17* has previously been shown to be involved in yeast DNA damage checkpoints *(14)*. The demonstrated role of this conserved checkpoint gene in IR-induced proliferation arrest and apoptosis confirmed the previously tentative conclusion that these are indeed bona fide checkpoint responses. Further, this result prompted experiments testing whether similar checkpoint defects could be elicited by RNAi of the *C. elegans* orthologs of other known yeast checkpoint genes. It was found that RNAi for worm orthologs of mammalian ATM and ATR, Rad-17, and p53bp1 indeed abrogated IR-induced proliferation arrest, further confirming the operation of conserved checkpoint pathways in this response *(13)*. However, defects in IR-induced apoptosis could be elicited only at a low penetrance, most likely because these checkpoint genes could only be partially inhibited in meiotic pachytene cells by RNAi *(13)*.

rad-5 was the first conserved checkpoint gene whose function in a DNA damage checkpoint was defined in the *C. elegans* system. *rad-5* is an essential gene, and the two known *rad-5* mutations result in temperature-sensitive lethality *(12)*. Cloning of *C. elegans rad-5* revealed that this gene is related to *S. cerevisiae TEL-2*, an essential gene shown to be involved in telomere-length regulation *(15)*.

HU-induced cell cycle arrest in the proliferating population of *C. elegans* germ cells also appears to be a bona fide checkpoint response, since the arrest is abrogated in the *rad-5* mutants *(12)*. The checkpoint pathway triggered by HU treatment is distinct from that triggered by IR treatment, however, since neither *mrt-2* nor *hus-1* appears to be required for HU-induced arrest.

In addition to checkpoint genes involved in both IR-induced proliferation arrest and cell death responses, one gene product has been demonstrated to play a role in triggering IR-induced apoptosis yet appears to be expendable for the proliferation-arrest response. Although it initially evaded detection by conventional homology searches, bioinformatics approaches using generalized profiles revealed that the worm genome encodes a distant homolog of the mammalian p53 tumor ssuppressor gene, termed *cep-1* (*C. elegans* p53-like) *(16,17)*. Sequence alignments revealed that many of the p53 residues implicated either in DNA binding or in oncogenesis are conserved in *cep-1*. Unlike mammalian p53 but similar to *Drosophila* p53, *cep-1* is not required for DNA damage-induced proliferation arrest *(16,17)*. The transcriptional activation of the *cep-1* target gene *egl-1* contributes in part to IR-induced germ cell death; thus the transcriptional induction of *egl-1* can also serve as a marker for DNA-damage checkpoint activation *(18)*.

2. Materials

1. M9 buffer: 3 g KH_2PO_4, 6 g Na_2HPO_4, 5 g NaCl, H_2O to 1 L, 1 mM $MgSO_4$ (added after sterilization); pH should be between 6.9 and 7.0.
2. NGM agar: 3 g NaCl, 17 g agar, 2.5 g peptone, 1 mL cholesterol (5 mg/mL in EtOH), 975 mL H_2O. Autoclave, and then add the following sterile solutions, mixing after each addition: 1 mL 1 M $CaCl_2$, 1 mL 1 M $MgSO_4$, 25 mL 1 M potassium phosphate (pH 6.0). Pour plates. Store in plastic boxes with covers at room temperature for a couple of days before use to allow the plates to dry.
3. 1X egg salts buffer: 118 mM NaCl, 48 mM KCl, 2 mM $CaCl_2$, 2 mM $MgCl_2$, 5 mM HEPES (pH 7.4).
4. PBT: 1X PBS (137 mM NaCl, 2.7 mM KCl, 10 mM Na_2HPO_4, 2 mM KH_2PO_4) plus 0.1% Tween-20.

3. Methods

3.1. Checkpoint-Mediated Germ Cell Apoptosis

The DNA damage checkpoint response during meiotic prophase is measured by scoring numbers of apoptotic germ cell corpses in the meiotic prophase region of the adult hermaphrodite germ line. Checkpoint mutants exhibit less germ cell death than wild-type worms, whereas repair mutants tend to exhibit increased levels of germ cell death (*1*). *C. elegans* germ cell deaths are similar to the programmed cell deaths that occur during somatic development of the nematode, and can be readily observed in living animals using standard Nomarski differential interference contrast (DIC) microscopy. Live worms are mounted for microscopy as follows (adapted from *19*).

3.2. Preparing Slides for Nomarski Microscopy

Prepare an agar pad as follows:

1. Place a slide between two spacer slides onto which you have put two layers of lab tape.
2. Put a few drops of hot 4% agar (in H$_2$O) on the slide.
3. Rapidly cover the hot agar with another slide and press down.
4. Let the agar solidify, then slide the top slide off the pad. Don't try to lift it off, but rather slide it off laterally.
5. Cut off excess agar on sides with razor blade.
6. Add 5 μL of 30 mM sodium azide in M9 buffer.
7. Add 5–30 worms.
8. Add coverslip.
9. Observe apoptotic corpses.

3.3. Morphology and Identification of Apoptotic Corpses in the C. elegans Germ Line

The method for quantifying the apoptosis response of the DNA damage checkpoint that requires the fewest experimental manipulations is direct observation in live animals by Nomarski microscopy. In order to use this approach, it is necessary to learn to identify apoptotic corpses in the germ line (*1*). Scoring is aided by the fact that germ cell apoptosis occurs mostly during the late pachytene stage, mainly at the bend region of the germ line (**Figs. 1** and **2**).

The first morphological sign of impending germ cell death is a decrease in the refractivity of the cytoplasm that occurs concomitant with an increase in refractivity of the nucleus (**Fig. 2B,** parts 1 and 2). In addition, a distinct boundary between dying cells and the surrounding germ line becomes visible (**Fig. 2A** "early corpse," and **Fig. 2B,** part 3); soon thereafter, both nucleus and cytoplasm become increasingly refractile and start to blend with each other until they resemble a flat, round, highly refractile disk (**Fig. 2A** "corpse," and **Fig. 2B,** part 4). After about 10–30 min, this flat disk often gets distorted and finally starts to disappear (**Fig. 2B,** parts 5 and 6). In late-stage corpses, the nucleus of the dying cell decreases in refractility, begins to appear crumpled, and finally vanishes within less than 1 h (**Fig. 2B,** parts 5 and 6). Late corpses often accumulate granular structures at their rim (**Fig. 2A** "late corpse"). The morphology of corpses as well as the kinetics of their disappearance is similar between somatic and germ cell apoptosis. However, as germ cells are only partially surrounded by a plasma membrane, the first step in germ-cell death is the full cellularization of the apoptotic cell. Under conditions where massive germ-cell death occurs, corpses tend to accumulate next to each other (**Fig. 2A**). Sometimes, when massive germ cell death occurs, "late apoptotic corpses" also accumulate at more proximal positions in the germ line and tend to align next to developing oocyctes (*see* **Note 1**).

3.4. Visualization of Germ Cell Corpses by Acridine Orange Staining

An alternative means for assessing germ cell apoptosis takes advantage of the fact that apoptotic corpses can be stained in live animals by acridine orange (AO) and visualized by fluorescence microsopy. Although this approach requires additional manipulation of the samples compared with Nomarski microscopy, it is preferred by some investigators.

1. Use 5 μL of AO stock (10 mg/mL) per mL of M9 as a staining solution; AO is light sensitive, so stock solution should be stored in dark tubes (AO: Molecular Probes Inc. A3568).
2. Add 0.5 mL of staining solution to 60-mm plate of worms.
3. Rotate plates to make sure that the staining solution is distributed evenly, and store plates in the dark for approx 1 h at RT.
4. Wash worms off plate with 1.5 mL M9 and transfer to a 1.5 mL tube. Spin worms down for 2 s at approx 800*g*; remove supernatant and wash three times in M9 by spinning for 2 s at 800*g* and removing the supernatant by aspiration.
5. Replate washed worms on new 60-mm plate and keep in the dark for approx 45 min.
6. Score worms with a fluorescence microscope within 1 h for the presence of fluorescent bodies indicative of apoptosis.

3.5. Regimens for Quantifying IR-Induced Germ Cell Death

To quantify apoptosis in response to IR treatment, the number of germ cell corpses is assessed following a range of radiation doses, at a range of time points following treatment. Two different regimens can be used; a most thorough investigation of potential mutants will employ both strategies. For both regimens, it is important that worms be closely age matched, which is accomplished by selecting hermaphrodite worms at the late L4 larval stage.

1. Irradiate late L4 animals with 0, 30, 60, and 90 Gy; score apoptosis after 12, 24, and 36 h (*see* **Note 2**).
2. Pick late-L4 animals, age 24 h, then irradiate with 0, 60, and 120 Gy; score apoptosis 2, 4, 6, and 12 h after irradiation (*see* **Note 3**)

Approx 15 germ lines should be scored for each time point and for each radiation dose. When different strains are to be compared, it is important to assess whether germ lines are of approximately equal size and proliferate similarly; in practice, egg-laying rates can be measured and used as a very rough surrogate for proliferation behavior (which is difficult to assess directly).

3.6. Assessing Checkpoint Activation by Scoring for Induction of egl-1

3.6.1. Transcripts

Induction of transcripts from the pro-apoptotic gene *egl-1* can also be used as an indicator of checkpoint activation *(18)*.

1. Synchronize worms and irradiate 24 h after the L4 stage.
2. Isolate total RNA 0.5–36 h postirradiation with RNAzol B (AMS Biotechnology) according to the manufacturer's protocol, treat with DNAseI, and further purify using the Rneasy kit (Qiagen).
3. For cDNA synthesis, reverse-transcribe purified total RNA with 250U of MultiScribe Reverse Transcriptase (Applied Biosystems) using random hexamer primers.
4. Estimate relative amounts of *egl-1* cDNA by quantitative PCR in an ABI Prism 7700 sequence detector system. For *egl-1* amplification, use the following two primers: 5'-CAGGACTTCTCCTCGTGTGAAGATTC-3' and 5'-GAAGTCATC GCACATTGCTGCTA-3', which span the single *egl-1* intron *(18)*. As an alternative to quantitative PCR, induction of *egl-1* transcription can be assessed qualitatively by using an *egl-1* GFP reporter*(18)*.

3.7. Assessing Mitotic Germ Cell Cycle Arrest Upon Ionizing Irradiation

1. To assess the proliferation arrest response to IR, worms are irradiated with 0–120 Gy at the late L4 larval stage.
2. 12 h postirradiation, mount worms for Nomarski microscopy and score the distal region of the germ line for the presence of sparsely spaced, enlarged nuclei.
3. Count the number of nuclei within a defined field *(1,12)*. The defined field used in several published studies corresponds to an area 3.125 μm × 6.25 μm in the most distal (premeiotic) region of the germ line **(Fig. 3)**; germ-cell nuclei in all focal planes are counted. Using this approach, <5 germ lines should be scored for each genotype and dose tested (*see* **Note 4**).

3.8. Assessing HU-Induced Germ Cell Proliferation Arrest

1. Prepare fresh plates (one plate/genotype assayed) for each chronic exposure experiment.
2. On standard 60 × 15 mm worm culture plates containing approx 12 mL of NGM agar *(20)*, spread a lawn of *E. coli* OP50 that fills most of the plate area. Prepare plates at least 2 d prior to applying HU (hydroxyurea), and let them dry on a benchtop (not in a humid box) at room temperature. For negative control, prepare plates without HU.

3. Overlay each plate with 250 μL of a solution containing 92 mg/mL HU (Sigma) in M9. Cover plates with their lids and allow solution to soak into plates overnight; use plates within 1 d (*see* **Note 5**).

4. Pick and add at least 40 L4 larvae of a given genotype to a single, freshly prepared HU plate. (As several worms in each experiment may die owing to a low level of general toxicity of HU, it is important to plate a number of worms in excess of the number to be dissected.) For controls, add L4 larvae of each genotype to non-HU-treated plates.

5. At 12 and 24 h following plating of worms on HU and control plates, prepare worms for DAPI staining. Transfer 10–20 worms into 30μL of 1X egg salts buffer on a 22 × 40 mm coverslip; sodium azide (15 m*M*) can be used as an anesthetic to immobilize worms, if desired. Use a single or a pair of 25-gage needles to quickly nick the worm, either in the vicinity of the posterior bulb of the pharynx, or in the vicinity of the anus. A successful nick will result in extrusion of one of the two gonad arms. Often a nick will only partially release the gonad arm; since full gonad release is required for the method of quantifying germ cell proliferation described below, at least five animals with a fully released gonad arm are required. Dissections must be performed quickly; dissected worms should spend no longer than 5 min in buffer prior to fixation.

6. Allow worms to settle briefly and carefully remove 15 μL of the buffer. Add 15 μL of fixation solution (7.4% formaldehyde [diluted freshly from a 37% solution] in 1X egg salts). Incubate dissected worms in fixative for 5–10 min.

7. Carefully remove 15 μL of the liquid, and sandwich worms/buffer/fix between the coverslip and a slide. SuperFrost Plus slides (Fisher) or lysine-coated slides should be used, as the internal tissue released from the worms sticks best to positively charged slides. Immediately immerse the slide, coverslip side up, in liquid nitrogen to freeze. Alternatively, place the slide on an aluminum block precooled to –70°C on dry ice. When frozen (approx 20 s), crack the coverslip off with a single downward slice of a razorblade situated between the edge of the coverslip and the slide itself. Immediately transfer the slide to 95% ethanol, prechilled to –20°C. Slides can be stored in this condition for at least 1 wk.

8. Warm slides to room temperature, then rehydrate through a series of 3-min PBT/ethanol washes containing increasing levels of PBT (1X PBS plus 0.1% Tween-20): for example, 25:75, 50:50, then 75:25 (PBT: 95% ethanol) followed by three washes in 100% PBT.

9. Incubate in 2 μg/mL 4', 6-diamidino-2-phenylindole (DAPI) for 5 min, then rinse five times for 5 min in PBT. Hold in the dark for 30 min to 1 h at 4°C in PBT; mount in 60% glycerol or alternative aqueous mounting media.

10. For scoring select only intact, fully released germ lines for analysis.

11. For consistent quantitation, germ lines should be "optically bisected" along the longitudinal axis of the gonad. Focus the microsope up and down through the Z-axis to reveal the rachis, the nucleus-deficient central cytoplasmic core of the germ line; the position of the rachis defines the bisection boundary. As it is often difficult to resolve nuclei on the side of the rachis farthest from the objective lens, it is best to restrict counts to nuclei in the half-volume of the germ line that

is closest to the objective lens (**Fig. 4C**). In the X and Y dimensions, count nuclei from the distal tip through the end of the pachytene region of the germ line, ending at the point where nuclei expand markedly in volume as chromosome condensation increases, reflecting transition into the morphologically distinct diakinesis stage of meiotic prophase (during which six separate highly condensed DAPI-stained bodies can be resolved in each nucleus). If properly age-matched, individual control animals should exhibit little variation (approx 15%) in the number of nuclei per gonad arm (e.g., **Fig. 4A**) (*see* **Note 6**).

3.9. Scoring for Radiation Sensitivity (Rad Assay)

Germ lines of worms defective either in checkpoint pathways or repair pathways typically exhibit hypersensitivity to IR. One easily assayed manifestation of such sensitivity is a severe drop in the production of viable progeny following genotoxic insult; this can be reflected in a drop on the number of zygotes produced, the fractional viability of the zygotes produced, or both. To enhance the accuracy of the assay the experiment is done in duplicates.

1. Irradiate late L4 larval worms with 0 Gy, 30 Gy, 60 Gy, and 120 Gy.
2. 24 h later, when the germ line is already fully developed, place five worms on worm plates that contain a freshly seeded bacterial lawn approx 1 cm in diameter at the center of the plate.
3. Remove adult worms from plates after 10–12 h, and determine the percentage of hatched embryos 24 to 36 h later.
4. Determine, the rate of egg-laying per worm per hour by adding the number of dead embryos and hatched larvae.

In a typical experiment, the lethality of wild-type animals is approx 30% and 70% after irradiation with 60 and 120 Gy, respectively.

3.10. Using RNAi and Co-Suppression to Inhibit the Function of Candidate Checkpoint Genes

Whereas detailed analysis of the role of a gene involved in the DNA damage response is best conducted using a permanent chromosomal mutation, in practice the potential involvement of candidate checkpoint genes will most often be assessed initially using posttranscriptional gene silencing (PTGS) methods to inhibit candidate gene function. Two approaches are available for use in the *C. elegans* germ line: RNAi methods, which deliver dsRNA molecules that direct the degradation of corresponding target mRNAs (*21*), and transgene-mediated co-suppression, whereby a high-copy transgene array elicits PTGS of the corresponding endogenous gene (*22,23*). (In the latter method, transgenes are *not* designed explicitly to express dsRNAs; the mechanisms of RNAi and cosuppression appear to be mechanistically related in that they have overlapping genetic requirements, but there are also distinctions.) Empirically, we have found that some genes respond more robustly to RNAi whereas others respond more robustly to co-suppression *(13)*; because the reasons for this are obscure at present, researchers particularly interested investigating the roles of a few specific genes are encouraged to try both approaches.

3.10.1. RNAi of Checkpoint Genes

dsRNA can be delivered to *C. elegans* by a variety of routes, including injection, soaking, and feeding. For the RNAi injection and soaking procedures, dsRNAs are produced by in vitro transcription and annealing of the complementary RNA strands. In the injection procedure, dsRNA is injected into the gonad or into the gut of adult worms *(21)*. In the soaking procedure, worms are incubated in a solution of dsRNA *(24)*. In the RNAi feeding procedure, the gene to be inactivated is cloned into an *E. coli* vector that allows for the inducible transcription of both DNA strands *(25)*. In practice, we have found that the delivery of RNAi by feeding has turned out to be the most successful technique for inactivating DNA damage checkpoint genes (Anton Gartner, unpublished observation). Further, it is easier to block IR-induced proliferation arrest than to block IR-induced apoptosis.

1. For RNAi by feeding, clone a cDNA or approx 1 kb of an exon-rich sequence into the L4440 RNAi feeding vector, which allows for inducible transcription of both strands of the insert, and transform into the HT115 *E. coli* strain.
2. Spread transformed *E. coli* on an LB amp plate overnight (2–3 cm^2). Resuspend the *E. coli* lawn in 200 μL LB, and use 50 μL of the resuspended culture to seed a NGM Amp (100 μL/mL) plate containing 6 m*M* IPTG.
3. Add, after a plate has dried, approx 3 P0 worms to the plate and incubate at 15°C for 3–4 d.
4. Three F1 worms (at the early L4 stage) are transferred, individually, each to its own plate freshly seeded by bacteria, and allowed to lay eggs for approx 24 h.
5. F1 worms are then removed and F2 worms are allowed to grow up to the L4 stage, treated with IR, and analyzed for radiation-induced cell cycle arrest as described above.

3.10.2. Co-Suppression of Checkpoint Genes

1. For checkpoint gene inactivation by co-suppression, amplify the promoter sequence and the first two exons of a target gene by PCR.
2. Phenol-chloroform extract PCR product and *rol-6* transformation marker *(23)*.
3. Coinject 50 ng/μL PCR product with an equal concentration of *rol-6* transformation marker *(23)*.
4. Select stable transformants according to standard procedures in the next two generations, and animals harboring the transgene array are analyzed for checkpoint responses as described above.

4. Notes

1. For quantification purposes, one does not follow the appearance and disappearance of corpses, but instead records a "snapshot" of the number of corpses present at a given time in each scored germ line (see below for dose/timing regimens). In practice, there is some subjectivity in scoring; whereas, the highly refractile corpses are readily recognized, "early corpses" and "late corpses" may not be recognized as consistently by all investigators. Thus, it is crucial that all genotypes, time points, and doses to be compared in a given analysis be scored by the same individual. Further, a novice in the field has to confirm that the structures being scored as corpses are indeed apoptotic corpses by verifying that they are not present in worms defective for the cell-death genes *ced-3* and *ced-4*, and/or that they stain with the dye acridine orange.

2. The advantage of this counting regimen is that it is easier to perform, and higher levels of germ-cell death are generally obtained. For example, upon irradiation with 120 Gy, an average of up to 25 corpses per germ line bend can be scored 36 h after irradiation. There is a potential complication in interpreting the results from this regimen, however. Whereas corpses scored 12 h after IR exposure (and likely most scored 24 h after exposure) would already have entered meiotic prophase at the time of irradiation, those scored at the 36 h timepoint would likely have been premeiotic at the time of exposure; these may have first undergone a transient cell cycle arrest, then recovered from arrest before entering meiotic prophase. Thus, differences in the kinetics of recovery, proliferation, or meiotic entry could potentially contribute to observed differences between strains in levels of programmed cell death.

3. Under this second counting regimen, it is clear that the programmed cell deaths scored directly reflect the response of cells that were already in the pachytene stage at the time of exposure. However, the numbers of apoptotic corpses detected are considerably lower when this regimen is employed. To sensitize detection of IR-induced cell death, germ cell apoptosis can be scored in strain backgrounds (e.g., *ced-1*) that are defective in the engulfment of apoptotic corpses; corpses persist for prolonged periods in such mutants, increasing the numbers of corpses that can be detected at any given time.

4. As an alternative to Nomarski, IR-induced proliferation arrest can also be visualized and quantified in fixed DAPI-stained germ lines as described below for the assessment of the response to HU-induced proliferation arrest. Although this approach requires several processing steps, it facilitates the scoring of experiments involving many samples, since fixation prevents asynchrony. Furthermore, the DAPI staining procedure permits detection of chromatin bridges and/or evidence for unequal mitotic chromosome segregation in mutants.

5. The final concentration of HU should be approx 25 m*M*. If plates contain more or less than 12 mL of NGM agar, adjust the amount of HU added accordingly.

6. If toxicity is observed with HU treatment, a lower concentration of HU (or a shorter exposure time) that still elicits arrest should be explored.

References

1. Gartner, A., Milstein, S., Ahmed, S., Hodgkin, J., and Hengartner, M. O. (2000) A conserved checkpoint pathway mediates DNA damage-induced apoptosis and cell cycle arrest in *C. elegans. Mol. Cell* **5,** 435–443.
2. Seydoux, G. and Schedl, T. (2001) The germline in *C. elegans*: origins, proliferation, and silencing. *Int. Rev. Cytol.* **203,** 139–185.
3. Gumienny, T. L., Lambie, E., Hartwieg, E., Horvitz, H. R., and Hengartner, M. O. (1999) Genetic control of programmed cell death in the *Caenorhabditis elegans* hermaphrodite germline. *Development* **126,** 1011–1022.
4. Keeney, S. (2001) Mechanism and control of meiotic recombination initiation. *Curr. Top. Dev. Bol.* **52,** 1–53.
5. Rinaldo, C., Bazzicalupo, P., Ederle, S., Hilliard, M., and La Volpe, A. (2002) Roles for *Caenorhabditis elegans rad-51* in meiosis and in resistance to ionizing radiation during development. *Genetics* **160,** 471–479.
6. Neufeld, T. P. and Edgar, B. A. (1998) Connections between growth and the cell cycle. *Curr. Opin. Cell Biol.* **10,** 784–790.
7. Weinert, T. A. and Hartwell, L. H. (1988) The *RAD9* gene controls the cell cycle response to DNA damage in *Saccharomyces cerevisiae. Science* **241,** 317–322.
8. Dasika, G. K., Lin, S. C., Zhao, S., Sung, P., Tomkinson, A., and Lee, E. Y. (1999) DNA damage-induced cell cycle checkpoints and DNA strand break repair in development and tumorigenesis. *Oncogene* **18,** 7883–7899.
9. Murakami, H. and Nurse, P. (2000) DNA replication and damage checkpoints and meiotic cell cycle controls in the fission and budding yeasts. *Biochem. J.* **349,** 1–12.
10. Rhind, N. and Russell, P. (2000) Checkpoints: it takes more than time to heal some wounds. *Curr. Biol.* **10,** R908–911.
11. MacQueen, A. J. and Villeneuve, A. M. (2001) Nuclear reorganization and homologous chromosome pairing during meiotic prophase require *C. elegans chk-2. Genes Dev.* **15,** 1674–1687.
12. Ahmed, S., Alpi, A., Hengartner, M. O., and Gartner, A. (2001) *C. elegans* RAD-5/CLK-2 defines a new DNA damage checkpoint protein. *Curr. Biol.* **11,** 1934–1944.
13. Boulton, S. J., Gartner, A., Reboul, J., et al. (2002) Combined functional genomic maps of the *C. elegans* DNA damage response. *Science* **295,** 127–131.
14. Ahmed, S. and Hodgkin, J. (2000) MRT-2 checkpoint protein is required for germline immortality and telomere replication in *C. elegans. Nature* **403,** 159–164.
15. Kota, R. S. and Runge, K. W. (1998) The yeast telomere length regulator *TEL2* encodes a protein that binds to telomeric DNA. *Nucleic Acids Res.* **26,** 1528–1535.
16. Schumacher, B., Hofmann, K., Boulton, S., and Gartner, A. (2001) The *C. elegans* homolog of the p53 tumor suppressor is required for DNA damage-induced apoptosis. *Curr. Biol.* **11,** 1722–1727.
17. Derry, W. B., Putzke, A. P., and Rothman, J. H. (2001) *Caenorhabditis elegans* p53: role in apoptosis, meiosis, and stress resistance. *Science* **294,** 591–595.

the mutants is unable to arrest the cell cycle in response to the drugs. Wild-type cells will arrest in mitosis as large budded cells with undivided nuclei, and retain high viability in response to the benzimidazoles, but checkpoint mutants lose viability rapidly and will continue into the subsequent cell cycle.

The assay for the spindle checkpoint in yeast is to determine whether cells arrest in response to benzimidazoles, to excess Mps1 expression, or to mutations that activate the spindle checkpoint. The benzimidazoles cause cells to arrest in the cell cycle because of two separable checkpoints—the kinetochore-dependent spindle checkpoint and the spindle orientation checkpoint. The kinetochore-dependent checkpoint arrests cells at the metaphase to anaphase transition, and the spindle orientation checkpoint arrests cells after anaphase is completed, when cells exit mitosis. There are different assays for the two transitions. The kinetochore-dependent spindle checkpoint arrests cells by inhibiting the activity of Cdc20, a specificity factor for the anaphase-promoting complex (APC/C). Mad2 binds Cdc20 to prevent the proteolysis of the mitotic inhibitor, Pds1 (securin), which is bound in a separate complex to a thiol protease, Esp1 (separase) *(5)*. When Cdc20 is active, separase is released as a result of proteolytic destruction of securin by the APC/C. Separase cleaves Mcd1/Scc1, a subunit of the cohesin complex that is responsible for maintaining cohesion between sister chromatids. The sister chromatids separate and cells enter anaphase. The metaphase to anaphase transition is assayed by determining the stability of Pds1, determining whether cohesion is maintained and whether sister chromatids separate. The exit from mitosis is assayed by determining the subcellular localization of Cdc14 and the stability of Clb2, a B-type cyclin that must be proteolyzed to assure DNA replication in the subsequent cell cycle. The Cdc14 phosphatase remains sequestered in the nucleolus, a kidney-shaped organelle associated with the nucleus, until the exit from mitosis. The release of Cdc14 triggers the APC/C-dependent proteolysis of Clb2. All reagents described in this chapter, especially strains containing mutations and epitope-tagged proteins, are readily available from individual researchers. The yeast research community is especially good at sharing strains and reagents. Complete methodologies for culturing yeast and for the essentials of yeast genetics are explained in *(8)*. Readers are referred to this source for information needed for constructing and propagating strains.

2. Materials

All materials are available from Sigma unless noted.

1. Anti-HA antibody: 12CA5 Mouse monoclonal anti-HA (Boehringer). Store at −20°C in 50% glycerol.
2. Anti-Myc antibody: 9E10 Mouse monoclonal anti-Myc (AbCAM). Store at −20°C in 50% glycerol.

3. Anti-mouse CY3-conjugated antibody: Goat anti-mouse IgG (Heavy and Light Chains) CY3-conjugated (Jackson ImmunoResearch).

4. Anti-mouse FITC-conjugated antibody: Goat anti-mouse IgG (Heavy and Light Chains) FITC-conjugated (Jackson ImmunoResearch).

5. Anti-mouse HRP-conjugated antibody: Peroxidase-conjugated AffiniPure Goat anti-Mouse IgG (Heavy and Light Chains) (Jackson ImmunoResearch Laboratories, Inc.), 0.8 mg/mL. Dilute 1:30,000 for use.

6. Benomyl (methyl 1-[butylcarbamoyl]-2-benzimidazole carbamate): Stock solution is 1.5 mg/mL in DMSO. Store at −20°C.

7. Bovine Serum Albumin Fraction V (BSA).

8. Chemiluminescent HRP detection reagent: SuperSignal Chemiluminescent Substrate for detection of HRP (Pierce).

9. Formaldehyde 37% solution.

10. Mating pheromone α-factor: WHWLQLKPGQPMY, molecular weight 1684. Prepare a 1×10^{-3} M peptide stock solution in water. Store aliquots at −20°C.

11. Media for yeast: YPD (Undefined) Medium (Yeast Extract, Peptone, Dextrose), SC (Synthetic Complete) Medium, SD (Synthetic Deficient) Medium.

12. MES: 0.5 mM MgCl$_2$, 1 mM EDTA, 1 M sorbitol.

13. Mounting medium: containing 1.5 μg/mL DAPI (Vector Laboratories, Cat. no. H-1200).

14. Multiwell slides (Carlson Scientific).

15. Nocodazole (methyl-[5-{2-thienylcarbonyl}-1h-benzimidazol-2-yl] carbamate: stock solution is 1.5 mg/mL in DMSO. Store at −20°C.

16. Normal Goat Serum (Vector Laboratories).

17. Paraformaldehyde-sucrose solution: 4% paraformaldehyde, 3.4% sucrose. Stable for several mo when stored at 4°C.

18. Phosphate-buffered saline (PBS): 10 mM sodium phosphate (pH 7.2), 0.9% NaCl. PBS/5% milk includes 5% nonfat dry milk, PBS/1% BSA includes 1% bovine serum albumin, PBS/normal goat serum includes 5 or 10% normal goat serum.

19. Pepsin solution: 50 mg pepsin, 550 μL 1 N HCl, 9.45 mL water.

20. Photo-Flo 200 (Kodak): working solution is 0.4% in water.

21. Poly-L-Lysine: solution is 0.1% in water. Store at room temperature.

22. Pronase: stock solution is 10 mg/mL in water. Store aliquots at −20°C.

23. Protein sample buffer: 0.06 M Tris-HCl (pH 6.8), 2% SDS, 5% glycerol, 0.0025% bromophenol blue, 4% β-mercaptoethanol. Prepare a 2X sample buffer, and just before use dilute with water and add β-mercaptoethanol.

24. Ribonuclease A (RNase A): use pancreatic RNase type 1-A, 5 times crystallized. The stock solution is 10 mg/mL RNase in 10 mN HCl. Boil for 30–60 min. Store at −20°C.

25. SCE: 1 M sorbitol, 20 mM EDTA, 10 mM Tris-HCl (pH 7.4).

26. Snap-cap 5-mL polystyrene tubes (Falcon).

27. Sodium citrate: 0.5 M sodium citrate in water, filtered. Dilute to 50 mM working stock.

28. Sonifier with micro tip (Branson Scientific).

29. Sorbitol-phosphate buffer: 1.2 M sorbitol, 0.1 M potassium phosphate buffer (pH 7.4).
30. SYTOX Green: 5mM in DMSO (Molecular Probes). Store in the dark at –20°C.
31. Zymolyase 100T: prepare 10 mg/mL stock in PBS. Store aliquots at –20°C (Seikagaku).

3. Methods

3.1. Assaying Response to Benzimidazoles

Benomyl is used in solid agar-containing medium and nocodazole in liquid medium (*see* **Note 1**). Dissolve both benomyl and nocodazole in DMSO and dilute to 1% DMSO in the medium.

1. Use medium containing benomyl at the sublethal concentration of 15 μg/mL to score sensitivity of strains. Spot serial 10-fold dilutions of cells onto plates and incubate at 23°C for 3–5 d. Wild-type cells have 95–100% plating efficiency. Mutants have less than 1% plating efficiency.
2. Medium containing 70 μg/mL of benomyl is fully restrictive for wild-type growth. Spread sonicated cultures of cells onto the surface of the plate and incubate at 23°C for 8 h. Over 90% of wild-type cells will arrest as large budded cells with two or four buds. Checkpoint mutants do not arrest and will re-bud, forming microcolonies of approx 10 cells.

Nocodazole is used in liquid medium at a concentration of 15 μg/mL in 1% DMSO. Wild-type cells will arrest as large budded cells. Cells can be assayed cytologically, biochemically, or by flow cytometry as described below.

3.2. Flow Cytometry

Flow cytometry is used to determine the status of DNA replication in a population of cells (**Fig. 1**). It is especially powerful when combined with cell synchrony to determine the kinetics of DNA replication and the length of cell cycle delay. Checkpoint-arrested haploid cells will accumulate with a G_2/M content of DNA and are distinctly different from cycling cells that have approximately equal proportions of cells with 1C and 2C contents of DNA. Cells lacking both kinetochore function and checkpoint function, or checkpoint mutants treated with nocodazole, will progress to the next cell cycle in the absence of DNA replication. Failure to segregate chromosomes will produce a distinctive population of cells with a 4C content of DNA.

Checkpoint mutants delay in the cell cycle in response to nocodazole *(6,7,9,10)*. The delay is eliminated in double mutants that lack both the kinetochore-dependent spindle checkpoint and the spindle orientation checkpoint *(9,10)*. This simple double mutant (epistasis) analysis is used to help determine whether a mutant belongs to one checkpoint pathway or the other.

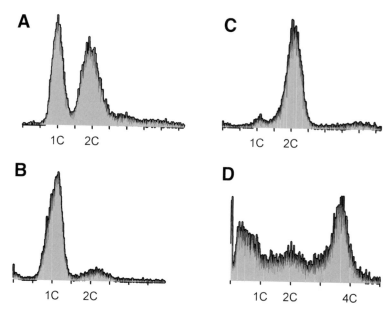

Fig. 1. Flow cytometry. (**A**) Wild-type cycling cells. (**B**) Wild-type cells arrested with α-factor. (**C**) Wild-type cells treated with nocodazole for 3 h. (**D**) Checkpoint mutant treated with nocodazole for 3 h.

1. Grow wild-type and mutant cells in liquid medium such as YPD to 10^7 cells/mL. If cell synchrony is required, arrest the cells with α-factor as described below. Add nocodazole to 15 μg/mL from a 1.5 mg/mL stock in DMSO. Add DMSO to control cells to give a final concentration of 1%.
2. Collect 1-mL samples of cells over time in plastic 5-mL snap-cap tubes, and fix by adding ethanol to a final 70%. Leave the samples at room temperature for 1 h. Cells can be stored for at least 1 wk in the 70% ethanol fixation solution at 4°C.
3. Wash the cells twice in 50 m*M* sodium citrate. Sonicate them in this buffer and resuspend in 2 mL of the same buffer containing 0.1 mg/mL of boiled pancreatic RNase.
4. Incubate the cells in the sodium citrate/RNase for 2 h at 37°C, then overnight at 4°C.
5. Centrifuge the cells (*see* **Note 2**) and resuspend them in 1 mL of pepsin solution for 5 min at room temperature.
6. Centrifuge the cells as before and resuspend them in 0.5 mL of 50m*M* sodium citrate containing 1 μ*M* Sytox Green. Stain the cells for 1 h at room temperature, then overnight at 4°C.
7. Analyze the cells by fluorescence microscopy, using a filter that emits in the red range (emission wavelength of approx 630 nm), to determine the efficiency of nuclear staining and RNase treatment (*see* **Note 3**).
8. Perform the flow cytometry analysis.

3.3. Cell Synchrony Using α-Factor

There are several ways to synchronize yeast cells, but the simplest, which does not require special equipment, is to use α-factor. *MATa* cells will arrest at START in the cell cycle in response to the 13-amino-acid polypeptide mating pheromone α-factor. *MATa* cells produce a protease (Bar1p) that destroys the peptide; therefore, successful use of α-factor in cell-synchrony experiments requires that you accommodate for Bar1p activity (*see* **Note 4**). The degree of synchrony can be determined by the unique pear-shaped (schmoo) morphology that α-factor-arrested cells adopt. There are three approaches.

1. Use low concentrations of cells (10^4/mL) and high concentrations of α-factor (3×10^{-6} M).
2. Use a higher concentration of cells (10^6/mL) in low-pH (3.5) growth medium, which inhibits the Bar1 protease, and use α-factor at 3×10^{-6} M. Adjust the pH of the medium with concentrated HCl.
3. Use *bar1* mutants that lack the protease. Cells can be used at a higher concentration (10^7/mL), with a low concentration of α-factor (3×10^{-8} M) (*see* **Note 5**).

Use complete (SC), synthetic (SD), or undefined (YPD) medium in all cases. Grow cells to the appropriate density and add the peptide directly to the medium (methods 1 and 3), or concentrate the cells, wash them in water, and resuspend them in fresh low-pH medium (method 2). Treat the cells with α-factor for sufficient time for the cells to complete approximately one and one-half cell cycles (approx 2 h at 30°C or approx 3 h at 23°C) (*see* **Note 6**). Assay cell morphology by phase-contrast microscopy to determine the arrest frequency. The presence of a schmoo, or mating projection, indicates arrest. Release the cells from α-factor arrest by washing them twice in water and resuspending them in medium containing 50 μg/mL pronase. Follow cell-cycle progression by noting the appearance of small buds, which occurs synchronously after approx 30 min of growth at 30°C. Greater than 80% of the cells should be arrested by pheromone and should be synchronous upon release (*see* **Note 5**).

3.4. Monitoring the Metaphase-to-Anaphase Transition

The spindle checkpoint inhibits two major transitions in the cell cycle: metaphase to anaphase and the exit from mitosis. There are simple molecular markers that are useful for distinguishing these events.

3.4.1. Sister Chromatid Separation

Follow the metaphase-to-anaphase transition cytologically by GFP tagging of individual loci on chromosomes. Two systems are employed.

1. Tet operator and GFP tet repressor fusion. An array of 112 Tet operators cloned into a yeast integrating plasmid, PRS306, are integrated at *URA3*. A Tet repressor–GFP fusion engineered for expression in yeast is integrated at *LEU2* (*11–14*). Wild-type cells treated with nocodazole will have a single spot of GFP fluorescence in the nucleus after arrest, corresponding to sister chromatids that remain in proximity owing to cohesion. Checkpoint mutants will have two dots of fluorescence, corresponding to separated sister chromatids. Synchronous cultures are used to determine the timing of sister chromatid separation.

2. Lac operator and GFP-lacI repressor fusion (**Fig. 2**). A similar approach is used with 256 tandem copies of the lac operator integrated on the arm of a test chromosome. A GFP-lacI fusion is integrated at a second locus (*11–14*). If the fusion is under the control of the *HIS3* promoter, it can be induced by preincubating the cells in medium that lacks histidine for 1 h prior to the beginning of the experiment to induce expression of the GFP-lacI fusion (*see* **Note 7**). As above, wild-type cells treated with nocodazole will arrest with a single spot of GFP fluorescence in the nucleus, and checkpoint mutants will have two dots, corresponding to separated sister chromatids.

3.4.2. Pds1 and Mdc1/Scc1 Turnover

Epitope-tagged Pds1 and Mcd1/Scc1 are routinely used to determine protein stability (*see* **Note 8**). Both proteins are molecular markers for the metaphase-to-anaphase transition because both are proteolyzed immediately before entry into anaphase. Pds1 is a substrate of the APC/C and is proteolyzed in a ubiquitin-dependent manner. The cohesin subunit Mcd1/Scc1 is a substrate of separase (Esp1). There are two approaches: the detection of protein turnover in individual cells by microscopy, or in populations of cells by Western blot. Both approaches are well suited for use with synchronous populations.

3.4.2.1. PDS1 TURNOVER BY MICROSCOPY

Detect Pds1 in cells by immunofluorescence following formaldehyde fixation. It is advantageous to have a strain with multiple epitopes fused to the protein of interest (such as 13-Myc or 6-HA) for optimal sensitivity (*see* **Note 8**).

1. Collect 1 mL of cell culture in mid-logarithmic growth (approx 1×10^7/mL). Add formaldehyde to cells in growth medium to a final concentration of 3.7% and incubate the samples at room temperature for 15–30 min to fix the cells (*see* **Note 9**).

2. Pellet the cells (30 s in a microcentrifuge, approx 11,000*g*), wash once with SCE, and resuspend in 1 mL of SCE. Briefly sonicate the cells (5–10 pulses) with the Branson sonifier using the 30% duty cycle, output level 2.

3. Add 5 μl of β-mercaptoethanol, 10 μL of 10 mg/mL zymolyase 100T, and incubate at room temperature for 10–35 min, assaying by phase-contrast microscopy (*see* **Note 10**).

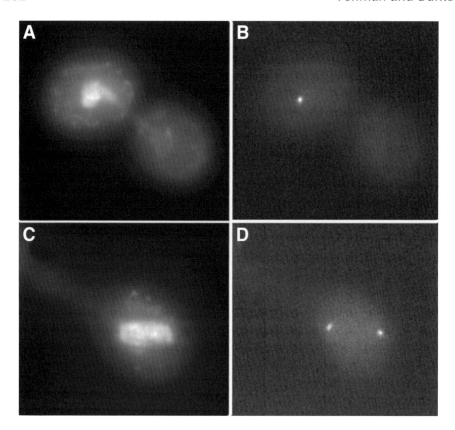

Fig. 2. Monitoring anaphase with LacI-GFP. DAPI stained cells (**A** and **C**) and GFP imaging (**B** and **D**). Wild-type cells (**A** and **B**) arrest in nocodazole with a single undivided nucleus and a single spot of GFP fluorescence because the sister chromatids are in proximity and cannot be resolved. A spindle checkpoint mutant does not arrest, and sister chromatids separate to produce two spots of GFP fluorescence.

4. Prepare a multiwell slide for the samples. Wash the slide in 1 N HCl for 15–30 min. Rinse the slide with distilled water, then ethanol. Air-dry the slide and put a 10μL droplet of poly-L-lysine on each well. Allow the slide to sit at room temperature for 10–20 min, and remove the excess poly-L-lysine with a micropipet or aspirator, leaving a thin liquid film across the well. Dry the slide thoroughly at 37°C (*see* **Note 11**) protected from dust, rinse it briefly in distilled water, and allow it to dry thoroughly again.

5. Pellet the zymolyase-treated cells in a microcentrifuge, approx 1300g (*see* **Note 2**), wash once in SCE, pellet again, and resuspend in SCE at 10–25% of the original cell culture volume.

6. Place 10 μL of cells in each well and allow 15 min for the cells to adhere. Remove loose cells with a micropipet or aspirator off to the side of the slide well and rinse the slides in PBS in a Coplin jar.

7. Place 10 μL of PBS/10% normal goat serum (*see* **Note 12**) on each well. Incubate the slide for 15 min at room temperature and remove excess solution with a micropipet.

8. Add 10μL of the appropriate primary antibody diluted in PBS/5% normal goat serum (*see* **Note 13**), to each well. Place the slide in a humidified chamber (such as a petri dish with a wet filter paper) for 1 h at 37°C, 2 h at room temperature, or overnight at 4°C.

9. Remove the antibody solution with a micropipet and rinse the slides in a Coplin jar for 5 min with PBS.

10. Add 10 μL of the secondary antibody, diluted in PBS/5% normal goat serum, to each well, and place the slide in a petri dish as in step 8. Incubate the slide for 1 h at 37°C.

11. Remove the antibody solution and rinse the slides with PBS for 5 min in a Coplin jar. Repeat this step.

12. Put a small droplet of mounting medium on each slide well, add a coverslip, and seal the edges of the coverslip with nail polish.

3.4.2.2. CHROMOSOME SPREADS FOR DETECTION OF McD1/Scc1

Mcd1/Scc1 is associated with chromosomal DNA from S phase until anaphase and then dissociates from the chromatin. To detect the dissociation, standard immunofluorescence is not appropriate, and chromosome spreads are used instead. The cells are simultaneously fixed, spread onto a glass slide, and cellular debris is extracted. The remaining DNA is subjected to immunofluorescence analysis. Therefore the assay is immunofluorescence colocalization of Mcd1/Scc1with DAPI-stained DNA (*see* **Note 14**).

1. Collect 1 mL of cells in mid-logarithmic growth (approx 1×10^7/mL). Pellet the cells, wash them once in sorbitol/potassium phosphate solution, and pellet again.

2. Resuspend the cells in 0.5 mL of the sorbitol/potassium phosphate buffer containing 5 μL of β-ME and 10 μL of fresh 100T zymolyase (10 mg/mL) per mL. Incubate the samples at room temperature. Monitor the zymolyase digestion by adding 1 μL of cells to 10 μL of 0.1% SDS and check for lysis by phase-contrast microscopy (*see* **Note 10**). Stop the reaction when 75–90% of the cells are spheroplasts (lacking cell walls) by gently spinning the cells (approx 1300*g*). Remove the digestion solution and resuspend the cells (gently) in 1 mL of cold MES. Gently pellet the cells again and resuspend them in 100 μL of MES.

3. Place 1 μL of spheroplasts on a clean, dry multiwell slide. Add 2 μL of paraformaldehyde/sucrose solution. Add 4 μL of 1% Lipsol, then 4 μL of paraformaldehyde/sucrose again. Allow a few seconds between each addition, vibrating the slide gently to mix the contents. At the end, spread the mixture gently across the entire well with a pipet tip. Let the slides dry overnight at room temperature.

4. Rinse the slide with 0.4% Photo-Flo 200 by brief immersion for 1 min. Submerge the slides in a Coplin jar with PBS for 10 min. Aspirate away the excess liquid and add a droplet of PBS/1% BSA to each slide well. Incubate at room temperature for 10–20 min.

5. Remove the PBS/1% BSA with an aspirator (off to the side of the wells), add droplets of primary antibody solution diluted in PBS/1% BSA (*see* **Note 13**), and incubate in a humidified chamber at room temperature for 1–2 h.

6. Rinse off the primary antibody with PBS and submerge in PBS in a Coplin jar for 5 min. Add the secondary antibody solution (in PBS/1% BSA) and incubate for 1 h in the humidified chamber at room temperature. Rinse off the antibody with PBS and wash twice in PBS in the Coplin jar for 5 min each wash.

7. Aspirate away excess liquid and add a small droplet (approx 1 µL) of mounting medium to each slide well, add a cover slip, and seal the edges with nail polish.

3.4.2.3. Pds1 and Mcd1/Scc1 Turnover by Western Blots

Analysis of Pds1 and Mcd1/Scc1 turnover is done with synchronous cells. Pds1 levels fall as cells enter anaphase as a result of proteolysis by the APC/C (**Fig. 3**). Pds1 degradation is assayed in individual cells by immunofluorescence, and in a population of cells by Western blot (*see* **Note 15**). Mcd1/Scc1 is proteolyzed by separase, and two breakdown products, 18 Kd N-terminal and 28 Kd C-terminal fragments, are generated (*see* **Note 16**). The final size that will be detected is dependent on the localization and nature of the epitope tag *(15,16)*. The size of the resulting peptide will be the sum of the Mcd1/Scc1 fragment and the epitope tag (**Fig. 4**).

1. Collect 1.5 mL of cells in mid-logarithmic growth at a density of approx 1×10^7/mL. Pellet the cells (30 s in a microcentrifuge, approx 16,000g).

2. Add 500µL of 0.1 N NaOH, vortex to resuspend the cells, and keep at room temperature for 5 min. Pellet the cells (30 s, approx 16,000g), and remove all of the NaOH solution (*see* **Note 15**).

3. Resuspend the cells in 100 µL of protein sample buffer, and heat the sample at 98°C for 5 min.

4. Pellet the cell debris (30 s, approx 16,000g), remove and save the supernatant.

5. Load approx 25 µg of total protein per lane on an SDS polyacrylamide gel.

6. Block nonspecific protein binding sites on the membrane with PBS/5% milk for 60 min at room temperature. Rinse the blot in PBS.

7. Dilute the primary antibody as required (*see* **Note 13**) in PBS/5% milk. The optimal concentration of primary antibody must be determined empirically. Incubate for 2 h at room temperature.

8. Wash the blot three times for 4 min each time in PBS, making sure to remove the PBS as thoroughly as possible after the last wash.

9. Add the HRP-conjugated secondary antibody, diluted in PBS/5% milk, and incubate for 1 h at room temperature.

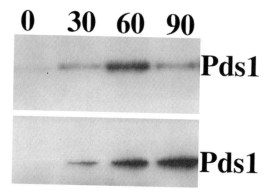

Fig. 3. Pds1-13Myc stability. Wild-type cells (lower row) and a spindle checkpoint mutant (upper row) were arrested with α-factor (0) and released into the cell cycle in the presence of 15 µg/mL of nocodazole. Samples were taken at the indicated times (minutes); proteins were extracted and processed for anti-Myc Western blots. Pds1 is absent in α-factor arrested cells but is stable and continues to accumulate in the wild-type cells. The checkpoint mutant cannot stabilize Pds1 and it turns over at 90 min.

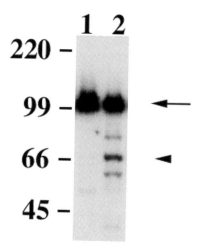

Fig. 4. Mcd1/Scc1 stability. Wild-type cells were synchronized with α-factor, released into the cell cycle, and samples were removed every 15 min and processed for Western blots. Full-length Mcd1/Scc1 (arrow) is detected in all samples, for example at 75 and 90 min after release into the cell cycle (lanes 1 and 2). The breakdown product is detected (arrowhead) only when the cells enter anaphase at 90 min (lane 2). Units are kD (kilodaltons).

10. Detect HRP with a chemiluminescence kit such as Pierce SuperSignal, following the manufacturer's instructions.

3.5. Monitoring the Exit From Mitosis

The exit from mitosis is monitored by the subcellular localization of Cdc14. The protein is localized in the nucleolus prior to the exit from mitosis. The protein can be detected in individual cells by immunofluorescence as described above for Pds1. A carboxy-terminal epitope-tagged version of Cdc14 with thirteen tandem Myc epitopes is used, and the protein is detected with the 9E10 monoclonal antibody. In addition, degradation of Clb2 protein indicates exit from mitosis. Clb2 stability is monitored using a 3-HA-tagged version of Clb2 and Western blots to follow populations of cells, as described for Pds1. The HA epitope is detected using the 12CA5 monoclonal antibody.

3.6. Obtaining Reagents

Request reagents such as strains and plasmids from individual researchers. Contact information is available at SGD, the *Saccharomyces* Genome Database (http://www.yeastgenome.org/).

4. Notes

1. Nocodazole loses efficacy as temperature is raised. Microtubule depolymerization, and consequently spindle checkpoint arrest, is fully effective for up to 3 h at 23°C. At 30°C, this effective arrest period is reduced to approx 2 h, and at 36°C to about 1 h. For experiments that must be done at the higher temperatures, one should perform spindle microtubule immunofluorescence and/or assay bud morphology to determine the effectiveness of the arrest.

2. Centrifugation at up to 16,000g for 30 s is appropriate for pelleting cells in all the protocols described here. Yeast cells can generally be pelleted by centrifugation at 1000–16,000g without negative consequences. This corresponds approximately to 3K–14K rpm in a typical microcentrifuge such as the Eppendorf 5415C. The only exception is that cells that have had their cell walls weakened by digestion with zymolyase should be pelleted at no more than 1500g.

3. Before performing the cytometry analysis, look at the samples with respect to the following: If the sonication and pepsin treatment worked properly, the cells should move individually and not be adherent to each other. If the RNase treatment and DNA staining have worked, the nucleus will be a distinct mass and there will be no cytoplasmic staining.

4. Depending on the nature of the experiment, give consideration to the use of *bar1* or *BAR1* wild-type strains. *bar1* strains arrest easily and efficiently (approx 95% G_1 cells), but release from the arrest less rapidly than *BAR1* strains. *BAR1* strains arrest with approx 85% G_1 cells, but they reenter the cell cycle rapidly. Both the arrest frequency and the release efficiency will affect the synchrony of the population. Assay bud morphology to determine arrest and release efficiencies. The schmoo is the characteristic elongated cell projection induced by exposure to mating pheromone. If the cell is unbudded or has a schmoo, it is in G_1 phase, and the initiation of budding indicates exit from G_1.

5. When beginning to work with a batch of α-factor, determine the minimum effective concentration of the peptide under the desired experimental conditions. Make serial dilutions of α-factor in water, use them to arrest cells, and determine arrest frequency. Cells will release from arrest most efficiently when the peptide is used at the minimum effective concentration. If release from arrest is inefficient, perform an extra wash before releasing the cells into growth medium.

6. It is useful to determine the cell cycle or doubling time of strains when beginning to work with them, particularly if they are mutants. This fundamental information will allow accurate prediction of the kinetics of growth, arrest, and release under specific experimental conditions. To make a growth curve, count cell density over a time course of logarithmic growth. Yeast cells will grow logarithmically in YPD (undefined medium) up to a density of 2×10^7 cells/mL and reach stationary phase at 2×10^8 cells/mL. Cells should be counted on a hemacytometer following sonication.

7. To optimize GFP signal from the LacO LacI-GFP chromosome tag, it is necessary to induce the *HIS3* promoter carefully. If necessary, increase induction time by keeping the cells in SC-His medium for up to several hours. Induction works well during a 2–3-h α-factor synchronization period. Adding 3-aminotriazole to the medium inhibits activity of the His3 enzyme imidazoleglycerol-phosphate dehydratase, inducing *HIS3* expression. 3 aminotriazole can be used at concentrations from 5 to 20 m*M* as required for adequate production of LacI-GFP. When using *ade2* mutants, supplement the SC-his medium with adenine to a final concentration of 20 mg/L to prevent the accumulation of a fluorescent product produced by the mutant. In an α-factor-arrested population, the frequency of cells with only one discernible GFP dot can be used as an indicator of arrest efficiency. Cells with two dots must have replicated that locus and are therefore not arrested in G$_1$. It is best to release α-factor-synchronized cells into rich medium, as this will promote rapid, consistent re-entry into the cell cycle. The amount of LacI-GFP fusion protein produced during induction is sufficient to give a detectable GFP signal throughout a time course of 5 h after release from the arrest.

8. The construction of epitope fusion proteins is a standard technique in yeast genetics *(8)*. These proteins are expressed from in-frame gene fusions of the epitope DNA sequence to the gene of interest. The number of immunoreactive epitopes present in the tag directly affects the sensitivity of detection of the fusion protein.

9. Fixation time is a key variable in yeast immunofluorescence. Some proteins, such as Pds1-13Myc, are best detected following 15–30 min of fixation, while others, such as tubulin, require 60–90 min of fixation for best detection. It may be necessary to optimize this parameter by trying various fixation times.

10. Zymolase digestion of cells must be done carefully for best immunofluorescence results. As cells progress through a time course of zymolyase treatment, the cell wall is broken down and made permeable, they lose their bright yellow appearance and become a dull light gray, then progress to darker gray. Cellular morphology also breaks down, and finally the cells become ragged and misshapen. Most procedures, such as Pds1 immunofluorescence, work well if the cells have

only been lightly digested. This also preserves cell morphology, which may be an important aspect of the data collection. Other procedures, such as chromosome spreading, benefit from longer digestion, as this allows more cellular debris to be removed by the subsequent extraction. If necessary, leave out the β-mercaptoethanol from the zymolyase reaction to make the digestion gentler.

11. To work properly, the poly-L-lysine must be allowed to dry completely on the slide. This will promote adhesion of the cells to the glass surface. When cells adhere properly, it should be possible to find anywhere from 10 to 100 cells in a single field of view on the microscope.

12. The PBS/10% goat serum or PBS/1% BSA are used to block nonspecific antibody binding. Goat serum is ideal for immunofluorescence applications in which the anti-mouse secondary antibody was generated in a goat host. Centrifuge all blocking and antibody solutions for 2–4 min at maximum rpm (approx $16,000g$) to remove aggregates and debris. Pipet from the top of the solution to avoid the debris.

13. Monoclonal antibodies to the HA and Myc epitopes both work very well for this type of immunofluorescence, as well as for Western blot analysis, although detection of Myc is sometimes better. Other antibodies, including antibodies to endogenous yeast proteins, also work. It is important to determine, by performing a dilution series, the optimal antibody concentrations to use for immunofluorescence or Western blotting. Here are some guidelines to begin with: For immunofluorescence, use the 12CA5 anti-HA at 4 μg/mL, and the 9E10 anti-Myc at 2 μg/mL. For Western blotting, use the 12CA5 anti-HA at 100 ng/mL, and the 9E10 anti-Myc at 50 ng/mL. The working antibody solutions should be diluted into the appropriate blocking buffer. For immunofluorescence, use PBS/5% normal goat serum or PBS/1% BSA. For Western blots, use PBS/5% milk.

14. This chromosome spread protocol is a scaled-down version of a previously described method *(17)*. This allows a time course of up to 12 samples to be mounted on a single multi-well slide. Since the samples are not fixed upon collection, it is important to take each time point sample through the zymolyase digestion process without delay, thereby preserving the kinetics of the time course. To be able to make meaningful comparisons of immunofluorescence signal strengths, optimize two key variables of the procedure: the time of zymolyase digestion, and fixation. Both affect the eventual distribution of the nuclear material on the slide surface. These variables should be optimized so that the nuclear material is spread evenly but not overly stretched along the slide surface. If the DNA mass is too widely spread, fluorescence signal will be weakened and difficult to quantify. Intensity of the fixation treatment will strongly affect the ability of the DNA to spread on the slide. Optimize fixation intensity by adding slightly more or less paraformaldehyde solution during preparation of the sample.

15. The protein sample preparation method used in the assay of Pds1 and Mcd1 stability was previously described *(18)* as a general method for preparation of *S. cerevisiae* protein extracts. It is important to remove the sodium hydroxide as completely as possible before adding protein sample buffer. This can be accomplished by thorough removal with an aspirator or by an additional brief wash in

PBS. Pds1 level is a reliable indicator of population synchrony during α-factor arrest. The protein is absent from G_1 cells, appearing only as the cells reenter the cell cycle.

16. Intact Mcd1 protein is abundant and easily detectable on a Western blot. However the degradation products, which indicate Esp1-dependent proteolysis, require longer exposures to be visible. If you are using chemiluminescence detection, be certain to rinse membranes thoroughly before adding the chemiluminescent reagent to remove all traces of sodium azide that might be in the antibody or blocking solutions.

References

1. Burke, D. J. (2000) Complexity in the spindle checkpoint. *Curr. Opin. Genet. Dev.* **10**, 26–31.
2. Nicklas, R. B. (1997) How cells get the right chromosomes. *Science* **275**, 632–637.
3. Cleveland, D. W., Mao, Y., and Sullivan, K. F. (2003) Centromeres and kinetochores. From epigenetics to mitotic checkpoint signaling. *Cell* **112**, 407–421.
4. Millband, D. N., Campbell, L., and Hardwick, K. G. (2002) The awesome power of multiple model systems: interpreting the complex nature of spindle checkpoint signaling. *Trends Cell Biol.* **12**, 205–209.
5. Yu, H. (2002) Regulation of APC–Cdc20 by the spindle checkpoint. *Curr. Opin. Cell Biol.* **14**, 706–714.
6. Hoyt, M. A., Totis, L., and Roberts, B. T. (1991) *S. cerevisiae* genes required for cell cycle arrest in response to loss of microtubule function. *Cell* **66**, 507–517.
7. Li, R. and Murray, A. W. (1991) Feedback control of mitosis in budding yeast. *Cell* **66**, 519–531.
8. Burke, D., Dawson, D., and Stearns, T. (2003) *Methods in Yeast Genetics. A Cold Spring Harbor Laboratory Manual.* 2000 Edition. Cold Spring Harbor Laboratory, Cold Spring Harbor, NY.
9. Li, R. (1999) Bifurcation of the mitotic checkpoint pathway in budding yeast. *Proc. Natl. Acad. Sci. USA* **96**, 4989–4994.
10. Alexandru, G., Zachariae, W., Schleiffer, A., and Nasmyth, K. (1999) Sister chromatid separation and chromosome re-duplication are regulated by different mechanisms in response to spindle damage. *EMBO J.* **18**, 2707–2721.
11. Straight, A. F., Belmont, A. S., Robinett, C. C., and Murray, A. W. (1996) GFP tagging of budding yeast chromosomes reveals that protein-protein interactions can mediate sister chromatid cohesion. *Curr. Biol.* **6**, 1599–1608.
12. Straight, A. F., Marshall, W. F., Sedat, J. W., and Murray, A. W. (1997) Mitosis in living budding yeast: anaphase A but no metaphase plate. *Science* **277**, 574–578.
13. Nabeshima, K., Nakagawa, T., Straight, A. F., et al. (1998) Dynamics of centromeres during metaphase-anaphase transition in fission yeast: Dis1 is implicated in force balance in metaphase bipolar spindle. *Mol. Biol. Cell* **9**, 3211–3225.
14. Minshull, J., Straight, A., Rudner, A. D., Dernburg, A. F., Belmont, A., and Murray, A. W. (1996) Protein phosphatase 2A regulates MPF activity and sister chromatid cohesion in budding yeast. *Curr. Biol.* **6**, 1609–1620.

15. Uhlmann, F., Wernic, D., Poupart, M. A., Koonin, E. V., and Nasmyth, K. (2000) Cleavage of cohesin by the CD clan protease separin triggers anaphase in yeast. *Cell* **103,** 375–386.

16. Uhlmann, F., Lottspeich, F., and Nasmyth, K. (1999) Sister-chromatid separation at anaphase onset is promoted by cleavage of the cohesin subunit Scc1. *Nature* **400,** 37–42.

17. Jin, Q., Trelles-Sticken, E., Scherthan, H., and Loidl, J. (1998) Yeast nuclei display prominent centromere clustering that is reduced in nondividing cells and in meiotic prophase. *J. Cell Biol.* **141,** 21–29.

18. Kushnirov, V. V. (2000) Rapid and reliable protein extraction from yeast. *Yeast* **16,** 857–860.

14

Purification and Analysis of Checkpoint Protein Complexes From *Saccharomyces cerevisiae*

Catherine M. Green and Noel F. Lowndes

Summary

The DNA damage-dependent checkpoint of *Saccharomyces cerevisiae* is a paradigm for eukaryotic checkpoint pathways that regulate cell cycle progression in the presence of insults to the genetic material. In order to better understand this pathway, we undertook a biochemical study of the proteins implicated in its functioning. Analysis of the hydrodynamic properties of a protein in a crude mixture can give insights into possible tertiary organization such as participation in high-molecular-mass protein complexes. We here describe the determination of Stokes radius and sedimentation coefficients for the Rad24 protein, which enabled us to predict that this protein was a component of a protein complex in crude yeast extracts. This led us to develop a protocol to purify this complex to homogeneity in order to determine the component proteins. The methods described here should be applicable to the hydrodynamic analysis and subsequent purification of any soluble protein from organisms amenable to genetic manipulation, such as yeast, as long as the function of that protein is not perturbed by the addition of an epitope tag.

Key Words: *S. cerevisiae;* DNA damage; checkpoint; purification.

1. Introduction

The DNA damage-dependent checkpoint pathway of *Saccharomyces cerevisiae* was the first to be identified *(1)*. This pathway delays the initiation of S phase, causes the slowing of S phase, and prevents the initiation and/or completion of mitosis if DNA damage is detected in the G1, S, or G2 phases of the cell cycle, respectively *(2,3)*. Activation of the checkpoint pathway also results in the transcription of DNA damage-responsive genes *(4)*. Initially, genetic approaches were used to identify components required for the functioning of this pathway, and many of the genes are highly conserved *(2,3)*. However, in order to fully dissect the pathway and to perhaps identify proteins

From: *Methods in Molecular Biology, vol. 280: Checkpoint Controls and Cancer, Volume 1: Reviews and Model Systems*
Edited by: Axel H. Schönthal © Humana Press Inc., Totowa, NJ

involved that also have other, essential cellular roles and so cannot easily be identified by genetic means, we undertook a biochemical study of the checkpoint proteins. We were encouraged to do this by our hydrodynamic analyses of these proteins in crude cell extracts, which suggested that they exist as components of multimeric complexes (unpublished observations).

We present methods for the determination of Stokes radius and sedimentation coefficients and for purification of checkpoint protein complexes in their native form from *S. cerevisiae*. These use a combination of traditional and affinity separations, and should be generally applicable. In particular, we have focused on the complexes containing Rad24 or Rad9 (*5,6*). These proteins are present at low copy number in growing *S. cerevisiae* cells (we estimate between 200 and 1000 molecules of each per haploid cell—unpublished observations) and so we engineered an epitope-tagged version of the protein of interest into the yeast genome under the control of the endogenous promoter. A schematic (not to scale) of the tagged Rad24 used and the main steps of the hydrodynamic analysis and purification procedure for Rad24 are outlined in **Fig. 1.** F1 This purification has allowed identification of the components of these complexes and analysis of their biochemical functions. These methods could theoretically be adapted for other low-copy-number proteins in yeast, as long as they tolerate the addition of an epitope tag somewhere on the surface of the molecule, typically at the amino or carboxyl terminus. It can also be adapted to purify proteins from crude extracts prepared from cells treated with physical or chemical agents, for example DNA damaging treatments, or from cells arrested at different points of the cell cycle.

2. Materials

All chemicals were from Sigma (Ultrapure) unless otherwise noted.

1. Yeast strain expressing the protein of interest with HIS and HA epitope tags (*see* **Note 1** and **Fig. 2**).
2. YPD medium: 1% yeast extract, 2% peptone, 2% glucose; sterilized by autoclaving. Store at room temperature.
3. Cell counter (e.g., Multisizer II, Beckman-Coulter).
4. BioFlo 5000 Fermenter (New Brunswick Scientific).
5. CEPA Z41 Continuous flow centrifuge (Carl Padberg).
6. Polyethylene 305-mm lay-flat tubing and heat sealer (Jencons).
7. Liquid nitrogen.
8. 2X lysis buffer: 300 mM KCl, 100 mM HEPES (pH 7.5), 20% glycerol, 8 mM β-mercaptoethanol, 2 mM EDTA, 0.1% Tween-20, 0.01% Nonidet P40; in H_2O. Store at 4°C. Add 4X protease inhibitors and 2X phosphatase inhibitors just prior to use.
9. 100X protease inhibitors: 25 µg/mL leupeptin, 125 µg/mL pepstatin A, 20 µg/mL PMSF, 30 mg/mL benzamidine, 125 µg/mL antipain, 80 µg/mL chymostatin (from a stock solution in DMSO); in ethanol. Store in aliquots at –80°C.

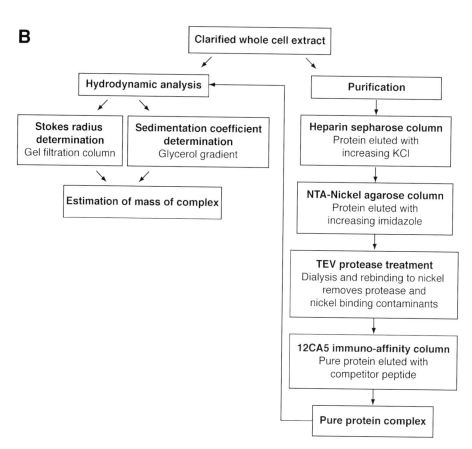

Fig. 1. Schematic showing the epitope tag requirements and an overview of the analysis and purification. (**A**) A yeast strain should be engineered to produce the protein of interest tagged with 10 histidines, an HA epitope, and an optional TEV cleavage site. The choice of N-terminal or C-terminal positioning will depend on the protein of interest. (**B**) The anticipated purification scheme. In the case of Rad24, the TEV protease cleavage step was not utilized, but this may be useful for other proteins.

10. 50X phosphatase inhibitors: 2 mg/mL NaF, 10 mg/mL β-glycerophosphate, 2 mg/mL Na_3VO_4, 20 mg/mL EGTA, 100 mg/mL sodium pyrophosphate; in H_2O. Store in aliquots at –80°C.
11. Ceramic pestle and mortar with 6.5-L capacity (Fisher Scientific).
12. Beckman 45 Ti rotor and Optima XL ultracentrifuge or similar.
13. Superose 6 PC 3.2/30 column and Smart chromatography system (Pharmacia).

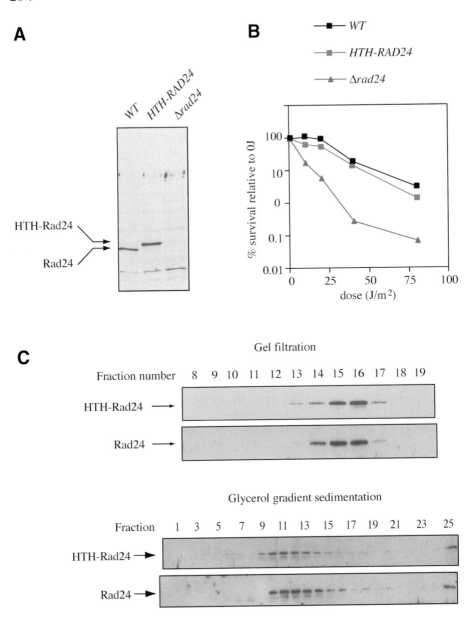

Fig. 2. The tagged protein retains biological function. (**A**) Western blot analysis was performed on equal quantities of crude extracts made from *W303*, *HTHRAD24*, or *rad24Δ* strains using an anti-Rad24 polyclonal antibody. The tagged protein is expressed at levels equivalent to the wild-type (WT) protein. (**B**) Analysis of the survival of *HTHRAD24* after UV irradiation compared to *W303* and *rad24Δ* strains. As determined by colony formation after UV irradiation, the *HTHRAD24* is not

14. Standard proteins of known Stokes radius and sedimentation coefficient (e.g., Gel Filtration LMW and HMW calibration kits [Amersham Pharmacia Biotech]).
15. 5-mL linear gradient former (Jencons).
16. 1X lysis buffer containing 20% glycerol: 150 mM KCl, 50 mM HEPES (pH 7.5), 20% glycerol, 4 mM β-mercaptoethanol, 1 mM EDTA, 0.05% Tween-20, 0.005% Nonidet P40; in H$_2$O. Store at 4°C. Add 2X protease inhibitors and 1X phosphatase inhibitors just prior to use.
17. 1X lysis buffer containing 35% glycerol: as above with 35% glycerol.
18. SW55 Ti swinging-bucket rotor (Beckman) or similar.
19. 400 mL heparin sepharose resin (Amersham Pharmacia Biotech).
20. Chromatography pump and fraction collector with UV and conductivity monitor (Biorad econosystem or similar) set up in cold room.
21. 30-cm column with 5-cm internal diameter and adapter (Bio-Rad).
22. 1X lysis buffer with 300 mM KCl and without EDTA: 300 mM KCl, 50 mM HEPES (pH 7.5), 10% glycerol, 4 mM β-mercaptoethanol, 0.05% Tween-20, 0.005% Nonidet P40; in H$_2$O. Store at 4°C. Add 2X protease inhibitors and 1X phosphatase inhibitors just prior to use.
23. 1X lysis buffer with 500 mM KCl and without EDTA: as above with 500 mM KCl.
24. 10 mL Ni-NTA superflow resin (Qiagen).
25. 20-cm column with 1-cm internal diameter and adapter (Bio-Rad).
26. 500 mM EDTA.
27. 1 M imidazole.
28. PBS (phosphate-buffered saline): 0.14 M NaCl, 3 mM KCl, 2 mM KH$_2$PO$_4$, 10 mM Na$_2$HPO$_4$; pH 7.4. Sterilize by autoclaving and store at 4°C.
29. Protein G sepharose (Amersham Pharmacia Biotech).
30. 12CA5 monoclonal antibody (Roche).
31. 0.1M borate buffer (pH 9.0): prepare a buffer from 0.1 M boric acid and 0.1 M sodium borate solutions, mixed in a ratio of 7:4, to give a buffer with pH 9.0.
32. Dimethyl pimelimidate (DMP). Purchased in 0.5 g aliquots, which should be stored desiccated at −20°C.
33. 1 M Tris buffer (pH 9.0): 0.76g Tris-HCl, 5.47g Tris base, in 50 mL H$_2$O.
34. 12CA5 competitor peptide (sequence KKKRILKMYPYDVPDYARIL).

3. Methods

The protocols below describe the production of crude cell extracts from large-scale *S. cerevisiae* cultures (**Subheading 3.1.**), followed the determina-

---

Fig. 2. *(continued)* significantly more sensitive to UV than WT, suggesting that HTHRad24 retains normal biological function. (**C**) Hydrodynamic analyses of Rad24 in extracts from *W303* and *HTHRAD24* strains. The hydrodynamic behaviors of the tagged and untagged proteins are not significantly different, suggesting that the tag does not perturb protein complex formation. Adapted from (**6**) with permission from Elsevier.

tion of hydrodynamic parameters (Stokes radius and sedimentation coefficient) of proteins within such extracts, using Rad24 as an example (**Subheading 3.2.**). This allows a determination of the molecular mass of the protein in its tertiary complexes. We then describe a procedure to purify Rad24 to homogeneity, which should be generally applicable to epitope-tagged proteins (**Subheading 3.3.**). Repetition of the hydrodynamic analysis on the purified material confirms that purification has not perturbed any protein complexes, and that determination of the polypeptide components of the purified material is relevant to the situation in crude extract.

3.1. Preparation of Large-Scale Yeast Whole-Cell Extracts (see Note 3)

1. Early in the day, pick a large, single colony of the required yeast strain (e.g., *HTHRAD24*, a *W303* derivative containing epitope-tagged *RAD24*, see **Note 1**) and grow for 10 h in 5 mL YPD medium in a 50-mL conical flask in an incubator at 30°C with agitation at 200 rpm.
2. Count the cell density (number of cells per mL) using a Coulter counter. Use this culture to inoculate 100 mL YPD in a 500-mL-capacity flask at the appropriate density so the culture will have a density of 1×10^7 cells/mL early the next day (*see* **Note 4**).
3. From this 100-mL culture, grow an 80-L culture to late log phase in a fermenter in YPD medium at 30°C (*see* **Note 5**).
4. Harvest the yeast cells by continuous-flow centrifugation (*see* **Note 6**). Wash the pellet twice in ice-cold water, and remove the liquid after each wash by centrifugation at 1000g in a standard large-capacity centrifuge. Weigh the pellet and note the weight (normally approx 600 g).
5. Make a bag from 30-cm polyethylene tubing double-sealed with a heat sealer. Leave one end open.
6. Transfer the yeast pellet to the bag using a flexible spatula or palette knife.
7. Cut a point from the end of the bag with scissors to leave a hole of approx 4 mm diameter. Fill a large, clean, plastic container with liquid nitrogen and extrude the yeast into the liquid nitrogen by squeezing the bag slowly. Continue until all the yeast is frozen as "spaghetti," topping up the liquid nitrogen as required (*see* **Note 7**).
8. Fill a 6.5-L-capacity ceramic mortar with liquid nitrogen (*see* **Note 8**). Add the yeast spaghetti. Use the mortar, wearing eye protection and insulating gloves, to carefully break up the spaghetti into smaller pieces.
9. Grind the yeast spaghetti until it is an extremely fine powder, similar to the consistency of talcum powder. This can take up to 2 h depending on the mortar, pestle, and starting quantity of yeast (*see* **Notes 9** and **10**). At all times maintain a small quantity of liquid nitrogen in the mortar.
10. An estimation of the amount of cell lysis can be obtained by smearing a little of the powder onto a slide, allowing it to defrost, and inspecting it with a microscope. The lysis is satisfactory when only a small proportion (10–20%) of intact cells remain, relative to ghosts (lysed cells) and debris (*see* **Note 11**).

11. To the mortar containing the yeast talc-like powder, add a volume of 2X lysis buffer equivalent to the initial mass of yeast used (i.e., 600 mL for 600 g). Add this in 50 mL batches, grinding into the yeast powder with the pestle.

12. When all the buffer has been added and a smooth powder obtained, the extract can be defrosted (or it can also be stored at –80°C for at least 2 wk prior to thawing). Transfer the powder to a clean beaker and let stand at room temperature until the extract is fully liquid (*see* **Note 12**). After defrosting, the extract should be maintained on ice at all times.

13. Remove unlysed cells and large debris by centrifugation at 1000g in a standard large-capacity centrifuge for 10 min at 4°C.

14. Clarify the extract by centrifugation of the supernatant from the low-speed spin at 186,000g in a Beckman 45 Ti rotor (or equivalent) for 1 h at 4°C.

15. Using a 25-mL pipet, remove and retain the supernatant from this step as clarified crude extract. It is important to exclude the upper lipid layer and the cloudy zone over the pellet (*see* **Note 13**). Determine the protein concentration using the Bradford assay. It should be between 20 and 40 mg/mL. We normally obtain approx 500 mL of clarified crude extract from one fermenter batch of yeast. This extract can be used directly for hydrodynamic analyses (**Subheading 3.2.**) or as the load for the heparin column (**Subheading 3.3.**), or frozen as 45-mL aliquots in 50-mL tubes in liquid nitrogen and stored at –80°C until used.

3.2. Hydrodynamic Analysis of Crude and Purified Complexes

3.2.1. Determination of Stokes Radius

1. Equilibrate a Superose 6 column on a Pharmacia "Smart system" with 1X lysis buffer with 300 mM KCl at a flow rate of 50 μL/min.

2. Pass 1 mL clarified crude cell extract (**Subheading 3.1., step 15**) though a 0.2-μm filter to remove particulate matter.

3. Inject 50 μL of this filtered extract onto the Superose 6 column using a 50-μL loop. Retain the rest for determination of the sedimentation coefficient (**Subheading 3.2.2.**).

4. Fractionate this material by running a further 3.2 mL of 1X lysis buffer with 300 mM KCl through the column. Collect 100-μL fractions. This procedure will separate the proteins in the extract according to their Stokes radius; proteins and protein complexes with a large Stokes radius will elute earlier from the column than those with a small Stokes radius. Remove a 10-μL aliquot of fractions 8 to 22 for analysis by Western blotting (an example is given in **Fig. 2**); flash-freeze the remainder and store at –80°C.

5. If the column is to be reused immediately, for example to calibrate with protein standards of known Stokes radius, or to determine the Stokes radius of the purified material (**Subheading 3.3.**), reequilibrate the column in 1X lysis buffer with 300 mM KCl. Otherwise wash thoroughly in water, then 20% ethanol, before storage.

6. The Stokes radius can be determined by comparing the elution position of the protein of interest to that of a selection of protein standards of known Stokes radius that have been fractionated on the same column in the same manner (*see* **Note 14**).

of the flow adapter as the column packs, leaving the smallest volume possible of buffer between the resin and the adapter.

4. Wash the column with 1 L of 1X lysis buffer with 150 mM KCl without protease or phosphatase inhibitors.
5. At a flow rate of 6 mL/min, pass 1 L of 1X lysis buffer with 500 mM KCL without protease or phosphatase inhibitors through the column to wash and pack.
6. Wash the column with 500 mL of 1X lysis buffer (150 mM KCl) without protease or phosphatase inhibitors.
7. Pass 500 mL 1X lysis buffer (150 mM KCl) plus protease and phosphatase inhibitors through the column at 6 mL/min.
8. Load 500 mL of the clarified extract onto the equilibrated column at 6 mL/min. Collect the flow through in case the protein does not bind to the column (*see* **Note 15**).
9. Wash the column at 6 mL/min with 500 mL lysis buffer containing 300 mM KCl and protease inhibitors but no EDTA (*see* **Note 16**). Collect 15-mL fractions throughout the wash.
10. Elute the protein at 6 mL/min with 1X lysis buffer containing 500 mM KCl and protease but no EDTA. Collect 15-mL fractions. After the purification the heparin sepharose should be regenerated (*see* **Note 17**).
11. Remove 50-µL aliquots from each fraction collected during steps 9 and 10 for analysis. Freeze the rest in liquid nitrogen and store at –80°C.
12. Analyze 5 µL of each fraction for the presence of the required protein by Western blotting and immuno-chemiluminescent detection. An example is given in **Fig. 3** (*see* **Note 18**).

3.3.2. Nickel Agarose Column

1. Pool the fractions from the heparin column containing the protein of interest, as the load for the nickel affinity column.
2. Transfer 10 mL bed volume of Ni-NTA resin (20 mL of a 50% slurry) to a 1-cm-diameter glass column, and wash with water at a flow rate of 1 mL/min to allow packing.
3. Equilibrate the resin with 50 mL 1X lysis buffer containing 300 mM KCl but no EDTA at a flow rate of 1 mL/min.
4. Add imidazole to the pooled heparin fractions to a final concentration of 20 mM.
5. Load the pooled heparin fractions (100–200 mL total) onto the nickel column at a flow rate of 1 mL/min. Retain the flow through. Monitor conductivity and UV absorbance throughout.
6. Wash the column with 20 mL 1X lysis buffer containing 300 mM KCl and 50 mM imidazole. Collect 1-mL fractions.
7. Elute the protein with 25 mL 1X lysis buffer containing 300 mM KCl and 250 mM imidazole but no EDTA. Collect 1-mL fractions.
8. Add EDTA to the fractions to a final concentration of 5 mM (*see* **Note 19**). Remove a 10-µL aliquot of each for analysis and flash-freeze the rest in liquid nitrogen before storage at –80°C.

9. Analyze each fraction for the presence of the required protein by Western blotting and immuno-chemiluminescent detection. An example is given in **Fig. 3** (*see* **Note 20**).

3.3.3. Preparation of Immunoaffinity Resin (see **Note 16**)

1. Resuspend 400 µL of a 50% protein G slurry in 15 mL PBS, centrifuge at 2000g, discard the supernatant, and repeat the PBS wash two more times.
2. Transfer the beads to a 1.5-mL microcentrifuge tube.
3. Add 0.625 mL purified 12CA5 antibody solution (*see* **Note 22**) and allow binding to occur for 30 min at 4°C with agitation.
4. Centrifuge the beads at 2000g, discard the supernatant, and wash the beads with 15 mL PBS, and then with a further 2 × 15 mL PBS.
5. Wash the beads twice in 15 mL of borate buffer, pH 9.0.
6. Remove a 0.5-g dimethylpimelimidate aliquot (DMP) from the freezer and dissolve in 50 mL 0.1M sodium borate. Check that the resulting solution has a pH above 8.5; if not, discard and remake with freshly made 0.1 M sodium borate. This DMP solution should be used immediately.
7. Covalently couple the antibody to the protein G beads by resuspending the washed beads in 15 mL of the DMP solution and incubating for 1 h at room temperature in a tube fixed onto a rotating wheel.
8. Wash the beads three times in pH 9.0 borate buffer.
9. Wash the beads once with 1 M Tris buffer pH 9.0, then incubate the beads in 15 mL 1 M Tris buffer pH 9.0 for 15 min at room temperature to block unreacted coupling sites.
10. Wash the beads twice in PBS and resuspend in PBS as a 50% slurry (*see* **Note 23**).

3.3.4. Immunoaffinity Purification

1. Defrost and pool the fractions from the nickel column that contain the protein of interest as determined by Western blot (**Subheading 3.3.2., step 9**).
2. Transfer 400 µL of the 50% 12CA5 bead slurry (**Subheading 3.3.3., step 10**) into a 15-mL tube and add 10 mL 1X lysis buffer with 300 mM KCl, including protease inhibitors and EDTA.
3. Centrifuge at 1000g for 3 min, remove supernatant, and resuspend beads in 10 mL 1X lysis buffer with 300 mM KCl, including protease inhibitors and EDTA. Repeat this wash.
4. Centrifuge the washed beads at 1000g and discard this final wash.
5. Resuspend the washed beads in the pooled peak fractions from the nickel column.
6. Allow binding to occur for 2 h at 4°C on a rotating wheel.
7. After binding, centrifuge at 1000g, remove and retain the supernatant, and wash the beads five times in 1 mL 1X lysis buffer with 300 mM KCl, including protease inhibitors and EDTA. Transfer the beads to a 1.5-mL microcentrifuge tube.
8. Elute the protein from the column by removing the final wash and incubating the beads at 30°C for 15 min in 200 µL 1X lysis buffer containing 300 mM KCl and 2 mg/mL 12CA5 competitor peptide.

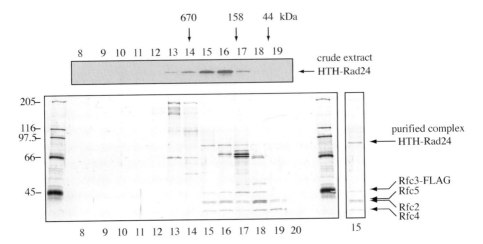

Fig. 4. Purification did not perturb the HTHRad24 complex. Comparison of the elution position from a Superose 6 gel filtration column of the crude material (upper panel—Western blot) and the purified material (lower panel—silver-stained gel) shows that the purified protein behaves like the starting material. In this case, the purification was from a yeast strain expressing a tagged version of RFC3 as well as HTHRad24, which explains why the pattern of bands seen in the purified material (lane 15) differs from that in lane E of **Fig. 3**.

9. Centrifuge the beads at 1000g, remove and retain the supernatant, which will contain the protein of interest; take a 5-µL aliquot for analysis, and flash-freeze the remainder in liquid nitrogen before storing at –80°C.

10. Repeat the elution step with a further 200 µL 1X lysis buffer containing 300 mM KCl and 2 mg/mL competitor peptide. Again, remove an aliquot of the supernatant and freeze the remainder.

11. Analyze the elution fractions for the presence of required protein by Western blot; if both contain protein they can be pooled. The protein can be used directly for functional assays and for hydrodynamic analysis to verify that the purification procedure has not disrupted the protein complex (**Subheading 3.2.**). However, if the protein concentration is too low for functional assays, or the final volume too great (e.g., if the entire sample is to be loaded onto an SDS-PAGE gel for mass spectrographic analysis), then continue with step 12.

12. To concentrate the protein, pool the elution fractions and add 20 µL Ni-NTA resin (previously equilibrated in 1X lysis buffer with 300 mM KCl, including protease inhibitors but no EDTA), and allow to bind for 1 h at 4°C. Proceed with either **steps 13–15** or **step 16**.

13. For functional assays and determination of hydrodynamic parameters, the protein can be eluted with up to 50 µL 1X lysis buffer containing either 150 or 300 mM KCl, protease inhibitors, and 250 mM imidazole. Small aliquots (1–5 µL) in

siliconized microcentrifuge tubes can be flash-frozen in liquid nitrogen and stored at –80°C.

14. Add 100 μL 1X lysis buffer with 300 m*M* KCl to 5 μL purified complex. Centrifuge at maximum speed at 4°C in a benchtop microcentrifuge.

15. Use 50 μL of the supernatant for determination of the sedimentation coefficient (as in **Section 3.2.2.**). Inject a further 50 μL of the supernatant onto a Superose 6 column and fractionate in 1X lysis buffer, to determine the Stokes radius, as for the crude extract (**Subheading 3.2.1.**). If the purification has not disrupted the protein complex, the hydrodynamic parameters should be unaltered. For an example *see* **Fig. 4**.

16. For a preparative gel before analysis by mass spectrometry, wash the beads from **step 12** three times in 1 mL 1X lysis buffer with 300 m*M* KCl. The proteins of interest can then be removed from the nickel column simply by boiling the resin in 20 μL acrylamide gel loading buffer (*see* **Note 24**). An example of a silver-stained gel showing the purified Rad24 material is given in **Fig. 3**.

4. Notes

1. The protocol described here is optimized for purification of Rad24 from the *HTHRAD24* strain. This strain was engineered from *W303* by homologous recombination *(7)* of a pRS303-based plasmid *(8)*, resulting in a tagged version of Rad24 being expressed from the endogenous Rad24 promoter (**Fig. 1**). Because a C-terminal tag had a destabilizing effect on Rad24 protein (Jorge Vialard, personal communication), the epitope tags were engineered at the N-terminal end of the polypeptide chain. Briefly, complementary oligonucleotides encoding ten histidine residues after a start codon were cloned into pRS303. The 1-kb genomic region immediately 5' of the *RAD24* start codon (this was assumed to contain the Rad24 promoter) was amplified by PCR and cloned before this His-encoding cassette. The first 1 kb of the *RAD24* open reading frame (ORF) (the smallest fragment that contained a unique restriction site in the resulting plasmid) was then amplified by PCR and cloned 3' of and in frame with the histidine encoding sequence. Complementary oligonucleotides encoding a linker sequence and a cutting site for the TEV (tobacco etch virus) protease *(9)* (*see* **Note 2**) and an HA epitope *(10)* were then cloned between the histidine encoding sequence and the Rad24 ORF. This plasmid was linearized with BsgI enzyme and used to transform *W303*. Integration events were selected on plates lacking histidine. Correct integration was verified by diagnostic PCR. The normal expression and presence of the epitope tags was verified by Western blotting (**Fig. 2**). The biological activity of the tagged protein was verified by analyzing the UV sensitivity of the *HTHRAD24* stain compared to *W303* (**Fig. 2**).

2. In the final purification procedure, the TEV cleavage step was omitted. There were many problems with this step in the case of Rad24, but it may be a useful addition if this procedure is attempted for the purification of other proteins (the protease is available from Gibco Life Technologies).

3. The protocol uses large quantities of yeast cells, as the proteins being investigated are of low abundance and furthermore are difficult to extract in soluble form. For more abundant proteins, the quantities can be scaled down accordingly. If a fermenter apparatus and continuous-flow centrifuge are not available, the large-scale protocol can still be performed by pooling batches of yeast cells grown on different occasions and processing them together at the extract preparation stage.

4. For example, using a strain with a doubling time of 90 min, a total of 2×10^6 (200 µL of a started culture with density 1×10^7 cells/mL) should be used for inoculation at 7:00 PM; the culture should then reach 1×10^7 cells/mL at 8:30 AM the next morning.

5. Late log for the *HTHRAD24* strain in this fermenter is around 7×10^7 cells per mL in YPD with extra glucose (4% final w/v). This strain has a doubling time of 90 min. The final density is achieved after around 22 h growth, starting from the appropriate quantity of seed culture. During the growth period, pH is maintained at 5.8 by the addition of 1 *M* NaOH as required.

6. The bowl of the centrifuge rotates at 20k rpm ($17,000g$). An 80-L culture is harvested in 35 min. The bowl is cooled by chilled water at 10°C.

7. The spaghetti can be stored at −80°C for many months if the purification is not to be performed immediately.

8. The mortar (not the pestle) is precooled at −80°C overnight.

9. A few muscular friends and some loud rock and roll are recommended at this stage!

10. Lysis of yeast cells in a coffee grinder in the presence of solid carbon dioxide has been described as an efficient way of producing high-quality extracts *(11)*. This method was found to result in severe aggregation artifacts for Rad24, but may be useful for other proteins.

11. Do not attempt to obtain complete lysis of the culture. Not only is this difficult, but we have found that it is possible to over-lyse the cells, leading to lower quality extracts with a much higher proportion of aggregated protein material.

12. It is essential to wait until the extract is completely thawed prior to centrifugation, as if ice pellets remain they will rise to the surface during the centrifugation.

13. Care should be taken at this stage. The clarified extract should be translucent and not at all turbid; if the strain used is *ade-* the resulting extract will be pink in color. It is preferable to discard a small proportion of the clarified extract than to contaminate it with lipids or material from the pellet. There is often a looser layer just above the main pellet, which should also be avoided.

14. The use of glycerol gradient sedimentation and gel filtration analysis gives both the sedimentation coefficient (SC) and Stokes radius (SR) of the protein complex when these procedures are performed with the appropriate size standards (e.g., ovalbumin SC 3.66×10^{-13} s, SR 3.05 nm; BSA SC 4.3×10^{-13} s, SR 3.55 nm; aldolase SC 7.35×10^{-13} s, SR 4.81 nm; catalase SC 11.3×10^{-13} s, SR 5.22 nm; thyroglobulin SC 18×10^{-13} s, SR 8.5 nm). The formula $M = (6\pi\eta Nas)/1-\upsilon\rho$ (where M = molecular weight, a = Stokes radius, s = sedimentation coefficient, υ

= partial specific volume, η = viscosity of medium, ρ = density of medium, and N = Avogadro's number) then allows estimation of the molecular mass of the complex. An assumed partial specific volume of 0.725 cm³/g is accurate for most proteins *(15)*. The viscosity and density of the medium are taken to be those of water, 1.002 × 10⁻² g/cm*s and 0.998 g/cm³, respectively. From our data the mass of the Rad24 complex is estimated to be approx 250 kDa.

15. A small aliquot of this material should be removed for analysis and the rest frozen in liqid nitrogen and stored at –80°C. After verification that the purification has been successful (e.g., by Western blot to check the protein of interest was properly retained on the column) it can be discarded.

16. EDTA was omitted, as the fractions may be used for the next step of the purification and this chelating agent is not compatible with nickel agarose.

17. Heparin sepharose should be regenerated after use by washing with 20 column vol of 0.1 *M* Tris-Cl (pH 8.5), 500 m*M* KCl; followed by 20 column vol of 0.1 *M* sodium acetate (pH 5.0), 500 m*M* KCl; followed by 20 column vol of 1X lysis buffer without protease inhibitors but with 0.02 % sodium azide. The column can be stored in this buffer at 4°C.

18. An approximately eightfold increase in the concentration of Rad24 relative to the total protein concentration was achieved on this column (data not shown).

19. This is in order to avoid nickel-mediated oligomerization *(12)*.

20. An approx 50-fold increase in the concentration of Rad24 relative to the total protein concentration was achieved on this column (data not shown).

21. This protocol is adapted from *(13)* and pp. 522–523 of *(14)*.

22. The stock concentration is 1.6 mg/mL. This results in a final ratio of 5 mg antibody to 1 mL beads.

23. With the addition of sodium azide at 0.02%, the beads can stored for up to 2 wk at 4°C.

24. This has the added advantage of removing a substantial proportion of the competitor peptide, which could otherwise interfere with the mass spectrographic analysis.

Acknowledgments

We would like to thank Jorge Vialard, Stephanie Kong, and Jesper Svejstrup for advice and the Cancer Research UK (formerly Imperial Cancer Research Fund) oligonucleotide synthesis, peptide synthesis, and fermenter suite services for valuable assistance. This work was initiated in the CDC laboratory at CRUK Clare Hall Laboratories, South Mimms, UK.

References

1. Hartwell, L. H. and Weinert, T. A. (1989) Checkpoints: controls that ensure the order of cell cycle events. *Science* **246,** 629–634.

2. Melo, J. and Toczyski, D. (2002) A unified view of the DNA-damage checkpoint. *Curr. Opin. Cell Biol.* **14,** 237–245.

3. Rouse, J. and Jackson, S. P. (2002) Interfaces between the detection, signaling, and repair of DNA damage. *Science* **297,** 547–551.